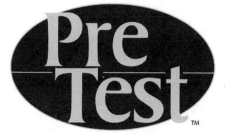

Physiology

PreTest™ Self-Assessment and Review

Notice

Medicine is an ever-changing science. As new research and clinical experience broaden our knowledge, changes in treatment and drug therapy are required. The authors and the publisher of this work have checked with sources believed to be reliable in their efforts to provide information that is complete and generally in accord with the standards accepted at the time of publication. However, in view of the possibility of human error or changes in medical sciences, neither the authors nor the publisher nor any other party who has been involved in the preparation or publication of this work warrants that the information contained herein is in every respect accurate or complete, and they disclaim all responsibility for any errors or omissions or for the results obtained from use of the information contained in this work. Readers are encouraged to confirm the information contained herein with other sources. For example and in particular, readers are advised to check the product information sheet included in the package of each drug they plan to administer to be certain that the information contained in this work is accurate and that changes have not been made in the recommended dose or in the contraindications for administration. This recommendation is of particular importance in connection with new or infrequently used drugs.

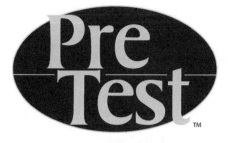

Physiology
PreTest™ Self-Assessment and Review
Eleventh Edition

James P. Ryan, Ph.D.
Professor and Associate Chair
Department of Physiology
Temple University School of Medicine
Philadelphia, Pennsylvania

Michael B. Wang, Ph.D.
Professor Emeritus
Department of Physiology
Temple University School of Medicine
Philadelphia, Pennsylvania

McGraw-Hill
Medical Publishing Division

New York   Chicago   San Francisco   Lisbon   London   Madrid   Mexico City
Milan   New Delhi   San Juan   Seoul   Singapore   Sydney   Toronto

The McGraw·Hill Companies

Physiology: PreTest™ Self-Assessment and Review, Eleventh Edition

2 3 4 5 6 7 8 9 0   DOC/DOC   0 9 8 7 6 5

ISBN 0-07-143653-7

This book was set in Berkeley by North Market Street Graphics.
The editor was Catherine A. Johnson.
The production supervisor was Phil Galea.
Project management was provided by North Market Street Graphics.
The cover designer was Li Chen Chang / Pinpoint.
RR Donnelley was printer and binder.

This book is printed on acid-free paper.

Library of Congress Cataloging-in-Publication Data

Physiology : PreTest self-assessment and review.—11th ed. / [edited by] James P. Ryan, Michael B.Wang.
    p. ; cm.
    Includes bibliographical references and index.
    ISBN 0-07-143653-7
      1. Human physiology—Examinations, questions, etc. II. Ryan, James P.
II. Wang, Michael B.
    [DNLM: 1. Physiological Processes—Examination Questions.
    2. Physiology—Examination Questions. QT 18.2 P578 2004]
    QP40 .P47 2004
    612'.0076—dc22   2004055929

Student Reviewers

Bobby Armin
University of California–Los Angeles
Los Angeles, California
Class of 2006

Frances Ford
Eastern Carolina University School of Medicine
Greenville, North Carolina
Class of 2004

Contents

Neurophysiology

Introduction

Each *PreTest™ Self Assessment and Review* allows medical students to comprehensively and conveniently assess and review their knowledge of a particular basic science, in this instance physiology. The 500 questions parallel the subject areas and degree of difficulty presented by the United States Medical Licensing Examination (USMLE) Step 1.

Each question is accompanied by the correct answer and its explanation. The explanation provides the reason why the correct answer is correct and, in many cases, the reason why the wrong answers are wrong. In addition, the explanation provides additional information relevant to the topic the question is designed to test. The references accompanying each question are from the major textbooks purchased by most medical students. The material in the referenced pages will provide a more expansive description of the subject matter covered by the question.

One effective way to use the PreTest™ is to answer 150 of the questions in two and a half hours. Write the answers on a separate sheet of paper and then compare your answers to the ones provided in the book. The PreTest™ can also be used as a review book. Answer a group of questions covering the same topic, check your answers, and then read the explanations and the referenced text pages. Whicheverp way you use the PreTest™, the most important part of your review is to be found in the explanations. The information in the explanations is designed to reinforce and expand on the material covered by the questions.

The High-Yield Facts found at the beginning of the book are not meant to be a complete list of all of the important facts, concepts, and equations necessary for understanding physiology. However, those that are included offer a solid foundation of the subjects they do cover and should be included in your review of physiology in preparation for a class test or for the Step 1 Examination. If you are not familiar with a section of the material presented in the High-Yield Facts, you should plan to do more reading. If, on the other hand, you have a good grasp of this material, you can feel confident in your knowledge of that topic.

Good luck on your exam.

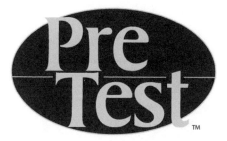

Physiology
PreTest™ Self-Assessment and Review

High-Yield Facts in Physiology

CELLULAR PHYSIOLOGY

- Ions, nutrients, and waste material are transported across cell membranes by diffusion, osmosis, and active transport.

Simple diffusion is described by the Fick equation. Carrier-mediated diffusion, called *facilitated diffusion,* is described by the Michaelis-Menton equation (see figure below).

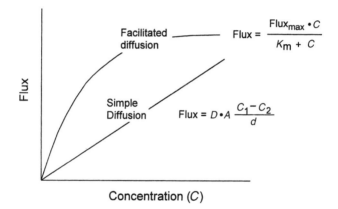

$$\text{Flux} = \frac{\text{Flux}_{max} \cdot C}{K_m + C}$$

$$\text{Flux} = D \cdot A \frac{C_1 - C_2}{d}$$

The flow of water through membranes by osmosis is described by the osmotic flow equation. Material dissolved in the water is carried across the membrane by solvent drag.

$$\text{Flow} = \sigma \cdot L \cdot (\pi_1 - \pi_2)$$

σ = reflection coefficient
L = hydraulic conductivity
π = osmotic pressure

The reflection coefficient (σ)

$$\sigma = 1 - \frac{P_{solute}}{P_{water}}$$

is an index of the membrane's permeability to the solute and varies between 0 and 1. Particles that are impermeable to the membrane have a reflection coefficient of 1. Particles that are freely permeable to the membrane have a reflection coefficient of 0.

The osmotic pressure (in units of mmHg) is calculated with the van't Hoff equation:

$$\pi = c \cdot R \cdot T$$

Cells shrink when placed in hypertonic solutions and swell when placed in hypotonic solutions. *Tonicity* is the concentration of nonpermeable particles. The following equation is used to calculate the steady state volume of the cell:

$$\pi_{initial} \cdot V_{initial} = \pi_{final} \cdot V_{final}$$

Active transport processes may be primary or secondary. Primary active transport processes, such as the Na-K pump, use the energy derived from the hydrolysis of ATP to transport materials against their electrochemical gradient. Secondary active transport processes, such as those that transport glucose and amino acids into renal or intestinal epithelial cells, use the energy from the Na^+ electrochemical gradient.

- All cells have membrane potentials. The magnitude of the membrane potential is determined by the membrane permeability and ion concentration gradient of the ions that are permeable to the membrane.

In the resting state, the membrane is primarily permeable to K^+, and, therefore, the resting membrane potential is close to the equilibrium potential for K^+.

The equilibrium potential is calculated with Nernst's equation:

$$\left(E_{ion} = -60 \cdot \log \frac{Conc_{in}}{Conc_{out}} \right)$$

The resting potential is calculated with the transference equation:

$$\left(\begin{array}{l} E_M = T_K \cdot E_K + T_{Na} \cdot E_{Na} \\ T_K = \dfrac{g_K}{g_{Na} + g_K}; \; T_{Na} = \dfrac{g_{Na}}{g_{Na} + g_K} \end{array} \right)$$

or with the Goldman equation:

$$E_M = -61 \cdot \log \frac{P_{Na} \cdot [Na]_{in} + P_K \cdot [K]_{in}}{P_{Na} \cdot [Na]_{out} + P_K \cdot [K]_{out}}$$

Action potentials are produced by voltage and time-dependent gates covering ion selective channels. Nerve and skeletal muscle membranes contain Na^+ and K^+ ion selective channels (see figure on p 3).

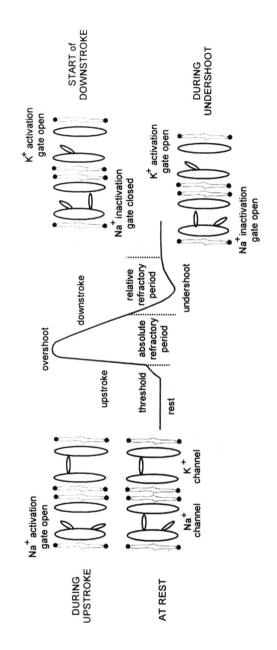

3

- Cardiac muscle membranes contain Na^+, K^+, and Ca^{2+} ion selective channels.
- The upstroke (phase 0) is produced by the activation of Na^+ channels.
- The initial repolarization (phase 1) is produced by inactivation of Na^+ channels.
- The plateau (phase 2) is caused by the activation of Ca^{2+} channels and the closing of inward rectifying (anomalous) K^+ channels.
- The downstroke (phase 3) is caused by the activation of the delayed rectifier K^+ channels and the inactivation of Ca^{2+} channels (see figure on p 5).
- Increasing extracellular K^+ concentration depolarizes the membrane and reduces its excitability. Excitability is reduced because the depolarization inactivates Na^+ channels. The reduced excitability can lead to muscle weakness and cardiac arrhythmias.
- Synaptic transmission is used to transmit information from one cell to another cell. The synaptic transmitter, released from the presynaptic cell by exocytosis, diffuses across a synaptic cleft and binds to a receptor on the postsynaptic cell. The effect produced on the postsynaptic cell depends on the identity of the synaptic transmitter and the receptor (see figure on p 6).

  Acetylcholine, which binds to the end plate of skeletal muscle cells, and glutamate and GABA, which bind to the postsynaptic membranes of many central nervous system membranes, open ion selective channels.

  Norepinephrine and acetylcholine, which bind to the postsynaptic membranes of smooth muscle cells, produce their effect by activating a G protein which, in turn, activates an enzyme-mediated response.

- Muscle contraction is produced by repetitive cycling of the myosin cross-bridges on thick filaments. The cross-bridges attach to actin molecules on the thin filaments and cause the thin filaments to slide over the thick filaments toward the center of the sarcomere (skeletal or cardiac muscle) or cell (smooth muscle; see figure on p 7).

  The initiation of contraction is called *excitation-contraction coupling*. In striated muscle, excitation-contraction coupling is initiated when Ca^{2+} binds to troponin. Troponin causes tropomyosin to move, thereby exposing the actin binding site to myosin (see figure on p 8).

  In skeletal muscle, Ca^{2+} is released from the sarcoplasmic reticulum (SR) when the muscle fiber depolarizes.

  In cardiac muscle, Ca^{2+} is released from the SR by the Ca^{2+} that enters the cell during the cardiac action potential.

  In smooth muscle, excitation-contraction coupling is initiated when Ca^{2+} binds to calmodulin.

  The Ca^{2+}-calmodulin complex activates myosin light chain kinase (MLCK) which, in turn, phosphorylates the 20,000-Da myosin light chains (LC_{20}). Cross-bridge cycling begins when the myosin light chains are phosphorylated.

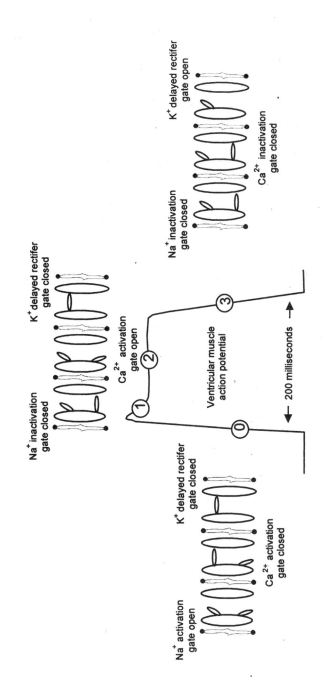

Na⁺ inactivation gate closed

K⁺ delayed rectifer gate closed

Ca²⁺ activation gate open

K⁺ delayed rectifer gate open

Na⁺ inactivation gate closed

Ca²⁺ inactivation gate closed

1

2

3

0

Ventricular muscle action potential

200 milliseconds

K⁺ delayed rectifer gate closed

Ca²⁺ activation gate closed

Na⁺ activation gate open

5

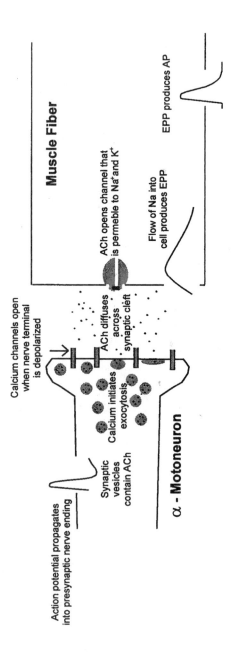

Muscle Fiber

ACh opens channel that is permeble to Na⁺and K⁺

EPP produces AP

Flow of Na into cell produces EPP

Calcium channels open when nerve terminal is depolarized

ACh diffuses across synaptic cleft

Calcium initiates exocytosis

Action potential propagates into presynaptic nerve ending

Synaptic vesicles contain ACh

α - Motoneuron

Receptor	Enzyme	Enzyme Effect	Postsynaptic Response
Adrenergic Alpha$_1$ (G$_o$)	Activation of phospholipase C	Formation of IP$_3$ and DAG	IP$_3$ releases calcium from SR DAG activates PKC
			Calcium activates arteriolar smooth muscle cells
Adrenergic Alpha$_2$ (G$_i$)	Inhibition of adenylyl cyclase	Reduction in cAMP formation	Relaxes GI smooth muscle cells
Adrenergic Beta (G$_s$)	Activation of adenylyl cyclase	Formation of cAMP	cAMP activates PKA which:
			• Increases Ca^{2+} entry into cardiac muscle cells and increases contractility • Increases sequestration of Ca^{2+} in bronchiole smooth muscle cells and relaxes muscle
Cholinergic Muscarinic (M$_1$)	Activation of phospholipase C	Formation of IP$_3$ and DAG	IP$_3$ releases calcium from SR DAG activates PKC
			Calcium activates GI smooth muscle cells

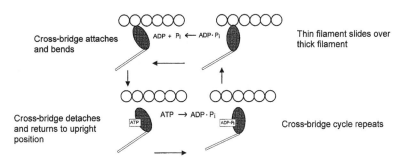

Cross-bridge attaches and bends

ADP + P$_i$ ← ADP·P$_i$

Thin filament slides over thick filament

Cross-bridge detaches and returns to upright position

ATP → ADP·P$_i$

Cross-bridge cycle repeats

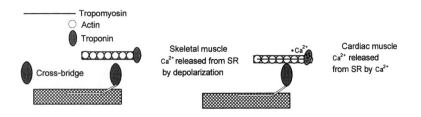

When dephosphorylated, the cross-bridges stay attached (or cycle slowly). The attached, slowly cycling cross-bridges are called latch bridges. Latch bridges allow smooth muscle to maintain force while minimizing energy expenditure.

CARDIAC AND VASCULAR PHYSIOLOGY

- The heart pumps the blood through the circulation. The cardiac output from the heart must be sufficient to perfuse all the organs and maintain a pressure adequate to perfuse the brain (see figure below).

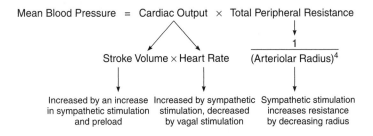

Cardiac output can be measured using the Fick equation:

$$CO = \frac{\dot{V}O_2 \text{ (oxygen consumption)}}{\text{(Arterial } O_2 \text{ content} - \text{Venous } O_2 \text{ content)}}$$

Resistance can be calculated using the Poiseuille equation:

$$R = \frac{8 \cdot \eta \cdot L}{\pi \cdot r^4}$$

η = viscosity
L = length
r = radius

Because resistance is inversely proportional to the 4th power of the radius, TPR is controlled by small variations in the diameter of the arterioles.

Blood pressure is maintained by the baroreceptor reflex, which responds to a decrease in blood pressure by increasing heart rate, contractility, and TPR, and by decreasing venous compliance.

Blood pressure decreases as blood flows through the circulation. The magnitude of the decrease is proportional to the resistance of each segment of the circulation. The greatest decrease occurs as blood flows through the arterioles. The segments of the circulation are in series with each other (see figure below).

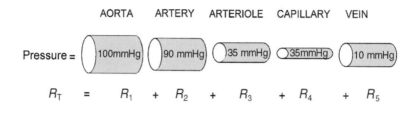

The quantity of blood flowing into each organ is inversely proportional to the relative resistance of each organ. For example, at rest approximately 20% of the cardiac output flows through the skeletal muscles. During exercise, when the resistance of the skeletal muscle vessels decreases, over 80% of the cardiac output can flow through the skeletal muscles. The organs in the body are in parallel with each other (see figure below).

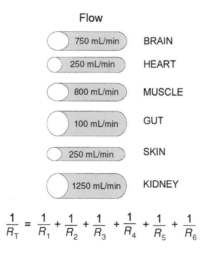

$$\frac{1}{R_T} = \frac{1}{R_1} + \frac{1}{R_2} + \frac{1}{R_3} + \frac{1}{R_4} + \frac{1}{R_5} + \frac{1}{R_6}$$

The velocity of blood through a vessel is proportional to the flow of blood through the vessel and inversely proportional to the area of the vessel:

$$v = \frac{Q}{A}$$

Increasing the velocity of blood can change flow from laminar (the fluid moves in a steady, orderly stream) to turbulent (the fluid movement is disorderly).

Turbulent flow produces a sound called a murmur if it occurs in the heart, or a bruit if it occurs in a blood vessel. Flow through stenotic or incompetent heart valves produces cardiac murmurs. Occlusion of blood vessels by a sclerotic plaque, for example, will produce bruits.

Turbulence can be predicted from Reynolds number:

$$N_R = \frac{\rho \cdot D \cdot V}{\eta}$$

ρ = density
D = diameter
V = velocity
η = viscosity

If Reynolds number exceeds 2000–3000, flow is likely to be turbulent.

- Stroke volume (and cardiac output) is dependent on preload, afterload, and contractility.

The relationship between preload and stroke volume (or cardiac output) is represented by a Starling curve. The Starling curve is shifted up and to the left by an increase in contractility or a decrease in afterload. The Starling curve is shifted down and to the right by a decrease in contractility or an increase in afterload (see figure below).

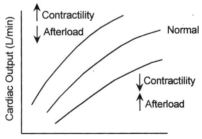

Preload is dependent on blood volume, venous compliance, and TPR. The relationship between these variables is represented by a vascular function curve. Changes in vascular volume or venous compliance cause a parallel shift in the vascular function curves. Changes in TPR cause the slope of the vascular function curve to change (see figure below).

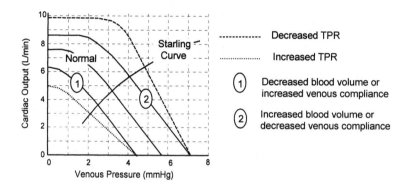

The change in pressure and volume within the heart during one cardiac cycle can be represented by a pressure-volume loop (see figure below).

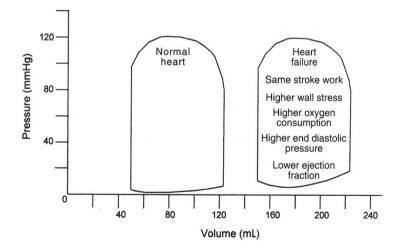

The work required to eject the blood is called the *stroke work*. The stroke work is the product of mean left ventricular systolic pressure and stroke volume:

$$\text{Stroke work} = \text{MLVSP} \cdot \text{SV}$$

Stroke work is equal to the area within the pressure-volume loop.

The energy required to eject the blood is dependent on the stroke work and the wall stress.

Wall stress is proportional to systolic pressure and the radius of the ventricle and inversely proportional to the thickness of the ventricular wall (law of Laplace):

$$\text{Wall stress} = \frac{P \cdot r}{\text{Thickness}}$$

Wall stress increases in heart failure because the preload increases to compensate for the decrease in contractility. The increased radius of the enlarged heart causes wall stress to increase, and, therefore, more energy is required to eject blood. If the coronary circulation cannot provide the necessary oxygen, ischemic pain (angina) results.

- Fluid exchange across capillaries is dependent on Starling forces:

$$\text{Filtration} = k_f \cdot [(P_{cap} + \pi_i) - (\pi_{cap} + P_i)]_i$$

Normally, the fluid filtered from the capillaries is returned to the circulation by the lymphatic system. Fluid accumulation in the interstitial space is referred to as *edema*.

Edema can result from:

An increase in capillary permeability, as during an inflammatory response

A decrease in plasma proteins, as during malnutrition

An increase in capillary pressure, as in heart failure (the increased end-diastolic pressure that occurs in heart failure causes the increase in capillary pressure)

A blockage of the lymphatic circulation

PULMONARY PHYSIOLOGY

- Air is moved in and out of the lungs by the movement of the diaphragm and chest. During inhalation, the diaphragm descends and the rib cage moves up and out. The expansion of the lungs creates a negative intra-alveolar pressure (with respect to atmospheric pressure) which draws air into the alveoli. The air moving into the lung with each breath is called the *tidal volume*. The amount of air moving into the lung per minute is called the *minute ventilation*.

Minute ventilation (V_{min}) = Tidal volume (V_T) · Breathing frequency (f)

At the end of inspiration, the air within the conducting airways is called the *anatomical dead space air* and does not contribute to gas exchange. The fresh air entering the alveoli each minute is called the *alveolar ventilation.*

Alveolar ventilation $(\dot{V}_A) = (V_T - V_D) \cdot f$

The physiological dead space is the sum of the anatomical and alveolar dead spaces. It is calculated with Bohr's equation:

$$V_D = V_T \cdot \left(\frac{F_{ACO_2} - F_{ECO_2}}{F_{ACO_2}} \right)$$

The anatomical dead space (in mL) is approximately equal to the weight (in pounds).

The alveolar dead space (areas of the lung that are ventilated but not appropriately perfused) is typically zero.

- The gas moving in and out of the lungs is measured with spirometry. Tidal volume is the gas moving in and out of the lungs with each breath. The maximum amount of gas that can be expelled from the lungs after breathing in as far as possible is called the *vital capacity.* The maximum amount of gas that can be expelled from the lungs after a normal breath is called the *expiratory reserve volume.* The maximum amount of gas that can be inhaled at the end of a normal breath is called the *inspiratory capacity.* The maximum amount of gas that can be inhaled at the end of a normal inspiration is called the *inspiratory reserve volume* (see figure below).

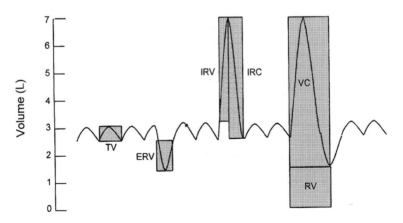

The gas remaining in the lung at the end of maximum expiration (the residual volume) cannot be measured by spirometry. It is measured using the helium dilution technique (see figure below).

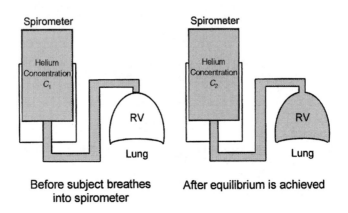

Before subject breathes into spirometer   **After equilibrium is achieved**

A known amount of helium is placed in a spirometer. The subject is connected to the spirometer when the volume in his or her lung is at the residual volume. After equilibration is achieved, the concentration of helium in the spirometer is measured. The following equation is then used to calculate the RV.

$$RV = V_{\text{Spirometer before equilibration}} \left(\frac{C_{\text{Spirometer before equilibration}}}{C_{\text{Spirometer after equilibration}}} - 1 \right)$$

The equation calculates whatever volume is in the lung when the subject begins to breathe into the spirometer. Therefore, the helium dilution technique can be used to measure any lung volume. For example, if the subject is connected to the spirometer at the end of a normal expiration, the FRC is calculated.

The FRC is the amount of gas in the lung at the end of a normal breath. It equals the RV + ERV.

The *total lung capacity* (TLC) is the amount of gas in the lung after a maximum inspiration. It equals RV + VC.

- The partial pressure of a gas is measured after water has been removed. Therefore, the partial pressure is calculated as a fraction of the atmospheric pressure remaining when the partial pressure of water vapor is subtracted.

$$F_{\text{gas}} \cdot (P_{\text{atm}} - P_{H_2O}) = F_{\text{gas}} \cdot (P_{\text{atm}} - 47 \text{ mmHg})$$

The average partial pressure of carbon dioxide in the alveoli is proportional to carbon dioxide production and inversely proportional to alveolar ventilation:

$$Fa_{CO_2} = (\dot{V}_{CO_2}/\dot{V}_a)$$

$$Pa_{CO_2} \propto (\dot{V}_{CO_2}/\dot{V}_a)$$

The average partial pressure of oxygen in the alveoli is calculated using the alveolar gas equation:

$$Pa_{O_2} = Pi_{O_2} - (Pa_{CO_2}/R)$$

$$R = (\dot{V}_{CO_2}/\dot{V}_{O_2})$$

R is the respiratory gas exchange ratio. Under normal circumstances its value depends on metabolism and is equal to 0.8. When the Pi_{O_2} is 100%, the value of R used in the alveolar gas equation is 1.0.

- The lung is an elastic organ that resists stretching. To expand the lungs, the inspiratory muscles must overcome the recoil force of the lungs and the resistance of the airways to airflow. The intrapleural pressure is a measure of the elastic and resistive work done by the inspiratory muscles. Expiration is usually passive. That is, the inspiratory muscles relax and the recoil force of the lungs expels the gas. Gas flow during expiration can be increased by contracting the expiratory muscles. However, the maximum expiratory flow is limited by airway compression (see figure below).

The work done by the lung can be represented by a pressure-volume loop. In restrictive airway disease (e.g., fibrosis), elastic work increases; in obstructive airway disease (e.g., asthma), resistive work increases (see figure on p 16).

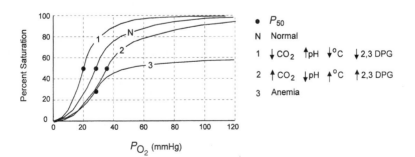

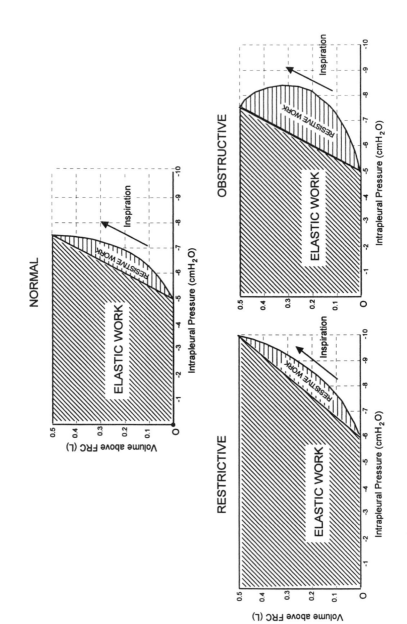

During active expiration, the alveolar pressure is the sum of the recoil force of the lung and the positive intrapleural pressure produced by the expiratory muscles. The intra-airway pressure decreases from the alveoli to the mouth. When the intrapleural pressure equals the intra-airway pressure (the equal pressure point) at a point along the airway where airway collapse can occur, increases in expiratory effort no longer increase expiratory flow (see figure on p 18).

Increases in lung compliance and/or increases in expiratory effort move the equal pressure point closer to the lung.

Maximum expiratory flow rates are lower in both obstructive and restrictive lung diseases.

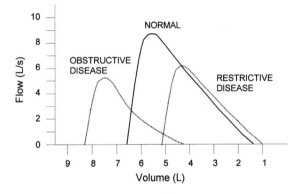

- Gas exchange across the alveolar-capillary membrane is very efficient. Under all but the most serious diffusion abnormalities (such as pulmonary edema), pulmonary capillary blood-gas tensions are in equilibrium with alveolar-gas tensions. Mixed venous blood returning from the systemic circulation has a PvO_2 of 40 mmHg and a $PvCO_2$ of 46 mmHg. Arterial blood has a PaO_2 of 95 mmHg and a $PaCO_2$ of 40 mmHg. The central chemoreceptors maintain $PaCO_2$ at 40 mmHg. The peripheral chemoreceptors will increase ventilation (and reduce $PaCO_2$ below 40 mmHg) if PaO_2 falls below 60 mmHg or if arterial pH is reduced by a metabolic acidosis.

  Most of the oxygen delivered to the blood is bound to hemoglobin (Hb O_2); a much smaller amount is dissolved in the blood. The amount of dissolved oxygen can be calculated if the PaO_2 is known:

$$\text{Dissolved } O_2 \text{ (mL } O_2/100 \text{ mL)} = 0.003 \cdot PaO_2$$

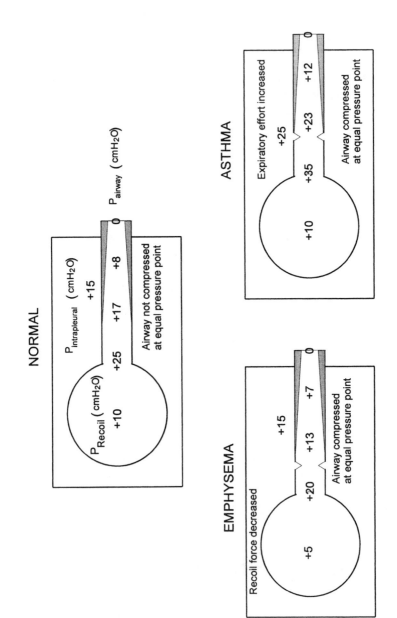

NORMAL

$P_{intrapleural}$ (cmH$_2$O)
+15
P_{Recoil} (cmH$_2$O)
+10   +25   +17   +8
P_{airway} (cmH$_2$O)
0
Airway not compressed
at equal pressure point

ASTHMA

Expiratory effort increased
+25
+10   +35   +23   +12   0
Airway compressed
at equal pressure point

EMPHYSEMA

Recoil force decreased
+15
+5   +20   +13   +7   0
Airway compressed
at equal pressure point

18

The amount of O_2 combined with hemoglobin can be determined from the oxy-hemoglobin saturation curve or, if the saturation of hemoglobin is known, can be calculated:

$$HbO_2 \text{ (mL } O_2/100 \text{ mL)} = \% \text{ sat} \cdot \text{g of Hb} \cdot 1.34$$

Hemoglobin is 97% saturated at the normal Pa_{O_2} (95 mmHg); 75% saturated at the normal $P\bar{v}_{O_2}$ (40 mmHg); and 50% saturated at 27 mmHg. The Pa_{O_2} at which hemoglobin is 50% saturated is called the P_{50}.

The hemoglobin saturation curve shifts to the right when P_{CO_2}, temperature, H^+ concentration, or 2,3-DPG concentration increases. Shifting the curve to the right makes it easier for O_2 to dissociate from hemoglobin in the tissues. Interestingly, CO causes the Hb saturation curve to shift to the left, making it more difficult for oxygen to dissociate in the tissues.

The $\dot{V}/\dot{Q}$ ratio affects the degree to which hemoglobin is saturated with oxygen.

The normal $\dot{V}_A$ of 4 L/min and cardiac output of 5 L/min produces a normal $\dot{V}/\dot{Q}$ ratio of 0.8. Areas of the lung with increased ratios are referred to as *alveolar dead space*; areas of the lung with decreased ratios are referred to as *intrapulmonary shunts*. Because areas of the lung with low $\dot{V}/\dot{Q}$ ratios cannot compensate for areas of the lung with high $\dot{V}/\dot{Q}$ ratios, the $\dot{V}/\dot{Q}$ ratio abnormalities result in low arterial P_{O_2} and lead to a large A − a gradient for oxygen (see figure below).

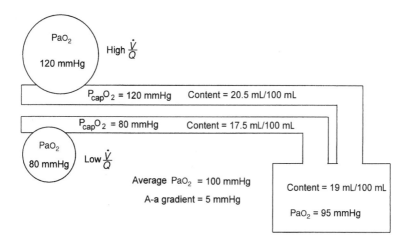

GASTROINTESTINAL PHYSIOLOGY

- The first stage in the digestion and absorption of food is chewing and swallowing. Chewing and swallowing can be initiated voluntarily or involuntarily. Chewing breaks food into small pieces and mixes them with salivary secretions. Swallowing is coordinated by a swallowing center in the brainstem. During the oral phase of swallowing, the tongue pushes the food into the pharynx; during the pharyngeal phase, peristaltic contractions and relaxation of the upper esophageal sphincter (UES) allow the food to enter the esophagus; during the esophageal phase, the lower esophageal sphincter (LES) relaxes and the food is propelled into the stomach by primary peristalsis. A secondary peristaltic wave, initiated by the presence of food in the smooth muscle, clears the esophagus of any food not propelled into the stomach by primary peristalsis.

- The stomach breaks food into small pieces and mixes the pieces with gastric secretions to produce a paste-like material called *chyme*. Liquids and chyme are forced through the pylorus by a rise in gastric pressure. Liquids empty from the stomach in one half-hour. Solids cannot pass through the pyloric sphincter until they are broken into small pieces (less than 1 mm^3), and, therefore, emptying of solids takes from 1 to 3 h.

Function	Gastric Functions	
	Orad Stomach	**Caudad Stomach**
Motility	Tone	
	Receptive relaxation	Trituration
	Accommodation	Emptying of solids
	Emptying of liquids	Reflux barrier
Secretion	HCl	
	Intrinsic factor	
	Mucus	Gastrin
	Pepsinogen	

Gastric emptying is slowed by the enterogastric reflex and the release of an inhibitory hormone called enterogastrone. The reflex and the secretion of enterogastrone are evoked by the presence of acid or fats in the duodenum.

The secretion of gastric acid by the parietal cells is regulated by paracrine (histamine), neural (vagus nerve), and hormonal (gastrin) influences.

- The intestine is responsible for the digestion and absorption of food and nutrients. During the digestive phase, food is slowly moved along the intestine by segmentation. During the interdigestive phase, the intestine is cleared of any nonabsorbed particles by the migrating motor complex.

Intestinal Phase of Digestion		
Stimulus	**Mediator**	**Response**
Partially digested nutrients	CCK	Pancreatic enzyme secretion
		Gallbladder emptying
		Decreased gastric emptying
	Enterogastrone and enterogastric reflex	Decreased gastric emptying
		Decreased gastric acid secretion
Acid	Secretin	Pancreatic/hepatic HCO_3^- secretion
		Decreased gastric acid secretion
Osmoles or distension	Enterogastrone and enterogastric reflex	Decreased gastric emptying
		Decreased gastric acid secretion

Sodium Transport Mechanisms in the Small Intestine			
Nutrient-Coupled Small intestine	Na^+/H^+ Exchange Jejunum	Neutral Ileum and colon	Electrogenic Colon

Functions of Small Intestine			
	Duodenum	**Jejunum**	**Ileum**
Motility	•	Segmentation (digestive period)	
		Migrating motor complex (interdigestive period)	
Secretion	CCK and secretin		HCO_3^-
Digestion		Intraluminal and brush border	
Absorption	Iron and folate	Folate	Bile acids and vitamin B_{12}
	⟵ Nutrients, water, and electrolytes ⟶		

Nutrient Digestion and Absorption		
Nutrient	**Digestion**	**Absorption**
Carbohydrates	Intraluminal (salivary, pancreatic amylase)	Active (glucose and galactose)
	Intestinal brush border enzymes	Passive (fructose)
Proteins	Intraluminal (gastric pepsin, pancreatic peptidases)	
	Intestinal brush border enzymes	Active (amino acids and di- and tripeptides)
	Intracellular (cytosolic peptidases)	
Lipids	Intraluminal (gastric and pancreatic lipase)	
	Bile salts required for micelle formation and solubilization of lipids	Passive
		Intracellular resynthesis
	Colipase essential for lipase hydrolysis of micellar lipids	Chylomicron formation

Fats, proteins, and carbohydrates are digested by intestinal enzymes. Bile is necessary for the digestion and absorption of fats. However, the amount of bile acids emptied into the proximal small intestine from the gallbladder is insufficient for complete fat digestion and absorption. Receptor-mediated active transport of bile acids in the terminal ileum returns the bile acids via the portal blood to the liver for secretion into the small intestine (this circulation of bile is called the *enterohepatic circulation*). Approximately 95% of the bile acid pool is recirculated from the intestine and about 5% is lost in the stool.

Water absorption is caused by osmotic forces generated by active sodium absorption. The source of water is both exogenous (oral input) and endogenous (GI tract secretion) and averages 8 to 10 L/day. Generally, less than 0.2 L/day is eliminated in the stool. The majority of water absorption occurs in the duodenum and jejunum. The colon exhibits a limited capacity to absorb water (4–6 L/day).

RENAL AND ACID-BASE PHYSIOLOGY

- The kidney is responsible for maintaining the constancy and volume of the extracellular fluid. The functional unit of the kidney is the glomerulus and its associated nephron. Each day, 160 to 180 L of fluid are filtered into the approximately one million nephrons in the human kidney. The glomerular filtration rate (GFR) is dependent on the Starling forces:

$$GFR = k_f \cdot [(P_{cap} + \pi_{BC}) - (\pi_{cap} + P_{BC})]$$

The amount of material filtered into the proximal tubule is called the *filtered load*. Approximately 20% of the plasma flowing through the glomerulus (RPF) is filtered into the proximal tubule:

$$\text{Filtration fraction} = \frac{GFR}{RPF}$$

The relative quantity of material excreted by the kidney (the renal clearance) is expressed as the volume of plasma that is completely cleared of the material by the kidney:

$$\text{Renal clearance} = (U_{conc} \cdot \dot{V})/P_{conc}$$

U_{conc} = Urinary concentration of material
P_{conc} = Plasma concentration of material
$\dot{V}$ = Urinary flow rate

If a material is filtered but not reabsorbed or secreted, its renal clearance will be equal to the GFR. The clearances of creatinine or inulin are used clinically to measure GFR.

If a material is completely cleared from the plasma during its passage through the kidney by a combination of filtration and secretion, its renal clearance will be equal to the RPF. The clearance of PAH is used clinically to measure RPF:

$$\text{Renal blood flow (RBF)} = \frac{RPF}{(1 - \text{hematocrit})}$$

- The proximal tubule is responsible for reabsorbing most of the material filtered from the glomerulus.

Material	% Reabsorbed	Mechanism
Na^+	60–70	Na/H exchange
		Na-nutrient cotransport
		Diffusion
K^+, urea, Cl^-	60–70	Diffusion and solvent drag
Glucose, amino acids	100	Na-nutrient cotransport
Phosphate	90	Na-nutrient cotransport
Bicarbonate	85	Indirectly via Na/H exchange

- The loop of Henle is responsible for producing a dilute filtrate. It reabsorbs approximately 25% of the salt and 15% of the water filtered from the glomerulus. The filtrate flowing from the loop of Henle to the distal convoluted tubule has a Na^+ concentration of approximately 100 meq/L.

- The distal nephron is responsible for regulating salt and water balance. Na^+ balance is regulated by aldosterone and atrial natriuretic peptide (ANP). Water balance is regulated by antidiuretic hormone (ADH), which is also called arginine vasopressin (AVP). K^+ balance is regulated by aldosterone.

  Aldosterone increases Na^+ reabsorption and K^+ secretion by the principle cells of the cortical and medullary collecting ducts. Aldosterone acts on the cell nucleus, increasing Na^+ conductance of the apical membrane (which, by allowing more Na^+ to enter the cell, increases Na^+ reabsorption), the number of Na^+-K^+-ATPase pump sites (which, by increasing intracellular K^+ concentration, increases K^+ secretion), and the concentration of mitochondrial enzymes.

  ANP decreases Na^+ reabsorption by the renal epithelial cells of the medullary collecting ducts.

  ADH increases water reabsorption by the principle cells of the cortical and medullary collecting ducts. ADH upregulates the number of water channels on the apical membrane of the epithelial cells by a cyclic-AMP-dependent process.

- The extracellular osmolarity is controlled by ADH.

  Increases in osmolarity stimulate the release of ADH from the posterior pituitary gland. ADH returns osmolarity toward normal by decreasing the amount of water excreted by the kidney. When osmolarity is decreased, ADH release is decreased and osmolarity is returned toward normal by increased water excretion.

  ADH also is secreted in response to low blood pressure. Under these conditions, reabsorption of water by the kidneys can make the extracellular fluid hypotonic.

- The extracellular volume is controlled by the salt content of the extracellular fluid. Salt content is controlled by aldosterone and ANP. Extracellular volume is monitored by low-pressure baroreceptors within the thoracic venous vessels and the atria and by pressure receptors within the afferent arteriole.

  Aldosterone secretion is controlled by the renin-angiotensin system. Renin is released from the juxtaglomerular cells (JG cells) in response to (1) decreased perfusion pressure within the afferent arteriole, (2) sympathetic stimulation of the JG cells, and (3) decreased Cl^- concentration in fluid bathing the macula densa. Renin catalyzes the conversion of angiotensinogen to angiotensin I. Angiotensin I is converted to angiotensin II (AII) by angiotensin-converting enzyme (ACE) located within the lung. AII stimulates aldosterone secretion from the adrenal cortex gland.

  ANP release is controlled directly by stretch receptors within the right atrium.

- Extracellular K^+ is controlled by aldosterone. Increases in extracellular K^+ stimulate the secretion of aldosterone, causing K^+ secretion to increase. K^+ transport into cells is increased by epinephrine and insulin.

- Each day, approximately 15,000 mmol of volatile acid (CO_2) and 50 to 100 meq of fixed acid (hydrochloric acid, lactic acid, phosphoric acid, sulfuric acid, etc.) are produced by metabolism. The pH of the extracellular fluid is maintained by buffering the acid as it is formed and excreting the acid over time. CO_2 is rapidly excreted by the lungs. The kidneys require approximately 24 h to excrete the fixed acids.

$$CO_2 + H_2O \xleftrightarrow{CA} H_2CO_3 \longleftrightarrow H^+ + HCO_3^-$$

When CO_2 is added to water, it forms H^+ and HCO_3^-.
The pH of plasma is calculated with the Henderson-Hasselbalch equation:

$$pH = 6.1 + \log \frac{HCO_3^-}{0.03 \cdot P_{CO_2}}$$

The H^+ concentration of the plasma is calculated with the Henderson equation:

$$H^+ = 24 \cdot \frac{P_{CO_2}}{HCO_3^-}$$

Plasma P_{CO_2} is normally maintained at 40 mmHg by the central chemoreceptors. Increases in P_{CO_2} cause an increase in ventilation; decreases in P_{CO_2} cause a decrease in ventilation. The respiratory system rapidly eliminates all of the CO_2 produced by metabolism.

Plasma HCO_3^- concentration is normally maintained at 24 meq/L by the kidneys. HCO_3^- is an important buffer for fixed acids produced by metabolism.

$$H^+ + HCO_3^- \longleftrightarrow H_2CO_3 \xleftrightarrow{CA} CO_2 + H_2O$$

The HCO_3^- lost during the buffering process is replaced by the distal nephron as the fixed acid (H^+ + anion$^-$) is excreted. The replaced HCO_3^- is called *new bicarbonate*.

The H^+ secreted into the urine is buffered by titratable acids (mostly phosphate) and ammonia. The following equation is used to calculate the net acid excretion:

$$\text{Net acid excretion} = ([\text{Titratable acids}] + [NH_4^+] - [HCO_3^-]) \cdot \dot{V}$$

- Acid-base disorders result from failure of the respiratory system and kidneys to maintain P_{CO_2} and HCO_3^- at their normal levels.

Disturbance	Examples	Compensation	Blood-Gas Profile	
Respiratory acidosis	Depression of the respiratory centers	Kidney produces new HCO_3^-	Pa_{CO_2} pH	↑ (cause) ↓ (result)
			HCO_3^-	↑ (compensation)
	Respiratory muscle fatigue			
Respiratory alkalosis	Hypoxemia, anxiety	Kidney excretes HCO_3^-	Pa_{CO_2} pH HCO_3^-	↓ (cause) ↑ (result) ↑ (compensation)
Metabolic acidosis	Excessive fixed-acid production, as in diabetes	Hyperventilation	HCO_3^- pH Pa_{CO_2}	↓ (cause) ↓ (result) ↓ (compensation)
	Failure of kidney to excrete H^+, as in renal tubular acidosis			
Metabolic alkalosis	Loss of acid, as in excessive vomiting	Hypoventilation	HCO_3^- pH Pa_{CO_2}	↑ (cause) ↑ (result) ↑ (compensation)
	Movement of H^+ into cells, as in hypokalemia			

NEUROPHYSIOLOGY

- Sensory receptors (touch, pain, temperature, smell, taste, sound, and sight) are activated by environmental stimuli. The stimulus produces a receptor potential; the magnitude of the receptor potential is proportional to the stimulus. The receptor potential produces a train of action potentials. Tonic receptors fire as long as the stimulus is present and encode intensity. Phasic receptors slow down or stop firing during the presentation of the stimulus and encode velocity.

- Sounds are detected by the hair cells within the organ of Corti of the inner ear. The organ of Corti consists of the hair cells and an overlying membrane called the tectorial membrane to which the cilia of the hair cells are attached. Sounds entering the outer ear cause the tympanic membrane to vibrate. Vibration of the tympanic membrane causes the middle ear bones (malleus, incus, and stapes) to vibrate, which in turn causes the fluid within the inner ear to vibrate.

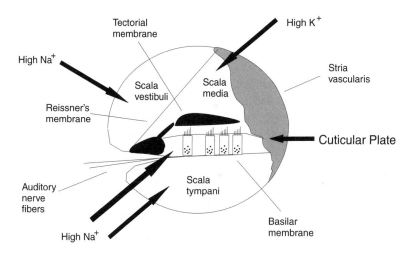

The inner ear is divided into three chambers (scala vestibuli, scala media, and scala tympani). The scala vestibuli is separated from the scala media by Reissner's membrane; the scala media and the scala tympani are separated by the basilar membrane. The stapes is attached to the membrane of the oval window, which separates the middle ear from the scala vestibuli. The scala tympani is separated from the middle ear by the round window. The organ of Corti sits on the basilar membrane. The fluid within the scala vestibuli and scala tympani (perilymph) is similar to interstitial fluid; the fluid within the scala media (endolymph) resembles intracellular fluid in that it contains a high concentration of K^+.

Vibration of the stapes causes the fluid within the scala tympani to vibrate, which in turn causes the basilar membrane to vibrate. Vibration of the basilar membrane causes the cilia to bend back and forth. Bending the stereocilia toward the kinocilium causes K^+ channels on the hair cells to open; bending the stereocilia away from kinocilium causes K^+ channels to close. Auditory hair cells are unusual because they are depolarized by the flow of K^+ into the cell. K^+ can flow into the hair cells because the endolymph surrounding the apical portions of the hair cells contains a high K^+ concentration.

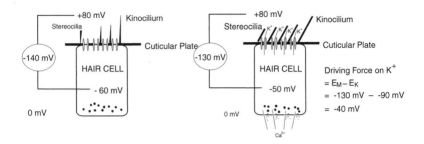

The basilar membrane is most stiff at the base of the cochlea (near the middle ear) and most compliant at the apex of the cochlea. High-frequency sounds cause a greater vibration of the stiff portion of the cochlea, and, therefore, the hair cells located near the base of the cochlea transmit information about high-frequency sounds to the auditory cortex. Similarly, low-frequency sounds are transmitted to the auditory cortex by the hair cells near the base of the cochlea, which are located on the more compliant portions of the basilar membrane.

- Light is detected by the rods and cones contained in the retina of the eye. The retina contains five types of neurons: photoreceptors (rods and cones), bipolar cells, ganglion cells, horizontal cells, and amacrine cells. Light rays from distant objects are normally focused on the photoreceptors by the cornea and the relaxed lens. When objects are brought closer to the eye, they are kept focused on the retina by the accommodation reflex, which causes the refractive power of the lens to increase. The rods and cones contain a visual pigment, called rhodopsin, which absorbs light energy. Rhodopsin contains two components: opsin, which determines the wavelength of light absorbed by rhodopsin, and retinal, which undergoes isomerization by light.

The photoreceptors are unusual because they hyperpolarize when they are stimulated by light. When the rods and cones are not stimulated, they are depolarized by the flow of Na^+ into the cell through Na^+ channels held in the open state by cGMP. The photoisomerization of retinal from its 11-cis form to its all-trans form activates rhodopsin, which in turn activates a G protein called transducin. Activated transducin activates a cGMP esterase. Hydrolysis of cGMP causes Na^+ channels on the rod and cone outer segments to close, which produces the membrane hyperpolarization.

The neurotransmitter keeps the bipolar cells and, therefore, the ganglion cells in a polarized and relatively quiescent state. Hyperpolarization of the photoreceptors stops the release of an inhibitory neurotransmitter, which in turn causes bipolar cells to depolarize. The bipolar cells stimulate ganglion cells, which in turn convey information about the light stimulus to the visual cortex. The ganglion cells are the only cells in the retina to produce an action potential. Their axons form the optic nerve.

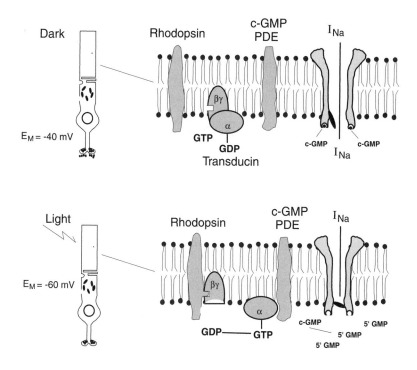

- Spinal reflexes provide rapid control of posture and movement. Ia afferents provide proprioceptive information about muscle length and velocity of movement. The sensitivity of the intrafusal muscle fibers is modulated by γ-motoneurons. Ib afferents provide proprioceptive information about strength of muscle contraction.

Name	Stimulus	Receptors	Afferent Fiber	No. of Synapses
Withdrawal reflex	Skin damage or irritation	Pain receptors (nociceptors)	Aδ and C	Polysynaptic
Stretch reflex	Muscle stretch	Intrafusal muscle fibers within muscle spindle	Ia	Monosynaptic
Lengthening reflex	Muscle contraction	Golgi tendon organ	Ib	Disynaptic

- Movement is initiated by the motor cortex. Motor commands reach the spinal cord through the pyramidal system (corticospinal tract) and the nonpyramidal system (corticoreticular and corticovestibular pathways). Lesions to the nonpyramidal system cause spasticity.
- The basal ganglia and cerebellum assist in the control of movement. Lesions to the basal ganglia produce paucity of movement or uncontrolled movements.

Disease	Possible Cause	Clinical Manifestations
Tardive dyskinesia	Dopamine antagonists used to treat psychotic diseases	Rapid, irregular movements (chorea) or slow, writhing movements (athetosis) of the face, mouth, and limbs
Parkinson's disease	Degeneration of the substantia nigra dopaminergic neurons	Tremor, paucity of movements, cogwheel rigidity
Huntington's disease	Degeneration of GABA-ergic neurons with the striatum	Chorea, ataxia, dementia
Hemiballism	Lesion of the contralateral subthalamic nucleus	Sudden flinging movements of the proximal limbs

- Lesions to the cerebellum produce uncoordinated movements.
- The vestibular system provides information about the position and movement of the head, coordinates head and eye movements, and initiates reflexes that keep the head and body erect. Lesions to the vestibular system result in loss of balance and nystagmus.
- The cortex is responsible for cognition, language, emotions, and motivation.

ENDOCRINE PHYSIOLOGY

- Most of the hormones secreted by the endocrine glands are controlled by the endocrine hypothalamus and pituitary gland. The posterior pituitary gland is divided into a posterior and an anterior lobe. The pituitary gland contains the axons of neurons located within the paraventricular and supraoptic nuclei of the hypothalamus. These hypothalamic neurons synthesize oxytocin (responsible for milk ejection and uterine contraction) and ADH (increases water permeability of renal collecting ducts). The anterior hypothalamus secretes six major hormones.

The synthesis and release of these hormones are controlled by the hypothalamus. The hypothalamic releasing hormones are secreted into the median eminence from which they enter the capillary plexus that coalesces to form the anterior pituitary portal veins. These veins form another capillary plexus within the pituitary from which the releasing factors diffuse to the pituitary endocrine cells.

- Thyroid hormone increases oxygen consumption and, therefore, the basal metabolic rate (BMR) by increasing the synthesis and activity of Na^+-K^+-ATPase. It acts synergistically with growth hormone to promote bone growth. Thyroid hormone is essential for proper development of the nervous system in newborn infants and for normal cognitive function in adults.

Pituitary Hormone	Hypothalamic Hormone Affecting Pituitary Hormone	Major Action of Pituitary Hormone
Thyroid-stimulating hormone (TSH)	Thyroid-releasing hormone (TRH)	Stimulates thyroid hormone synthesis and secretion
Adrenocorticotropic hormone	Corticotropin-releasing hormone (CRH)	Stimulates adrenocortical hormone (ACTH) secretion
Growth hormone	Growth hormone–releasing hormone	Synthesis of somatomedins by liver, which, in turn, stimulate protein synthesis, organ and bone growth
	Growth hormone inhibitory hormone (somatostatin)	
Follicle-stimulating hormone (FSH)	Gonadotropin-releasing hormone (GnRH)	Spermatogenesis (males) Estradiol synthesis (females)
Luteinizing hormone (LH)	Gonadotropin-releasing hormone (GnRH)	Testosterone synthesis (males) Ovulation (females)
Prolactin	Prolactin-inhibiting factor (dopamine) Thyroid-releasing hormone (TRH)	Breast development and milk production

- Adrenocortical steroid hormones (glucocorticoids and adrenocorticoids) are synthesized from cholesterol. Glucocorticoids promote gluconeogenesis, inhibit the inflammatory immune responses, and are essential for the vasoconstrictive action of catecholamines.

- Insulin and glucagon are secreted by the pancreas. Insulin affects carbohydrate, lipid, and protein metabolism in adipose, liver, and muscle tissues. Insulin is secreted by the β cells of the islets of Langerhans. Insulin increases the entry of glucose, amino acids, and fatty acids into cells. It promotes the storage of these metabolites and inhibits their synthesis and mobilization. Glucagon is secreted by the α cells of the islets of Langerhans. Glucagon's effects oppose those of insulin.

Cellular Physiology

Questions

DIRECTIONS: Each question below contains several suggested responses. Select the **one best** response to each question.

1. Which of the following characteristics of an axon is most dependent on its diameter?

a. The magnitude of its resting potential
b. The duration of its refractory period
c. The conduction velocity of its action potential
d. The overshoot of its action potential
e. The activity of its sodium-potassium pump

2. A 62-year-old male presents to the emergency room with an acute onset of aphasia and hemiparesis. A CT scan reveals an increase in intracranial fluid. Which one of the following solutions will be most effective in reducing intracranial pressure following a large hemispheric stroke?

a. 150 mmol sodium chloride
b. 250 mmol glycerol
c. 250 mmol glucose
d. 350 mmol urea
e. 350 mmol mannitol

3. An 82-year-old woman is brought to the emergency room complaining of extreme thirst and generalized weakness. She has consumed a large amount of orange juice to quench her thirst. Laboratory analysis reveals a significant hyperkalemia. Which one of the following changes in nerve membranes will most likely be observed?

a. The membrane potential will become more negative
b. The sodium conductance will increase
c. The potassium conductance will increase
d. The membrane will become more excitable
e. The Na-K pump will become inactivated

4. A 65-year-old male on digoxin for atrial fibrillation is told by his physician to get a blood analysis for K^+ on a regular basis because hypokalemia will increase his risk of digitalis toxicity. Hypokalemia increases the risk of digitalis toxicity because

a. The membranes of cardiac muscle cells are hyperpolarized
b. The intracellular potassium concentration of red blood cells increases
c. The excitability of nerve cells is increased
d. The inhibition of the sodium-potassium pump is increased
e. The amplitude of nerve cell action potentials is increased

5. A 35-year-old woman having an anxiety attack collapses. The EMT who arrives on the scene notes that she is hyperventilating and suspects that she is suffering from tetany, a continuous contraction of skeletal muscle fibers caused by an increase in the excitability of nerves and muscle membranes. The increased membrane excitability is caused by

a. Decreased release of inhibitory neurotransmitter from nerve terminals
b. Depolarization of the nerve and muscle membranes
c. Spontaneous release of calcium from the sarcoplasmic reticulum (SR)
d. Activation of sodium channels at more negative membrane potentials
e. Increased magnitude of the action potentials invading nerve terminals

6. A 72-year-old female presents to the emergency room with generalized weakness. An ECG reveals peaked T waves. Correcting which one of the following electrolyte disturbances will return the ECG to normal?

a. Hyperkalemia
b. Hyponatremia
c. Hypercalcemia
d. Hyperchloremia
e. Hypermagnesemia

7. The diagram below illustrates the concentration of a substance in two chambers. If the concentration of the substance in chamber A doubles, the diffusion of the substance will change from 10 mg/h to

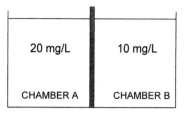

20 mg/L	10 mg/L
CHAMBER A	CHAMBER B

a. 5 mg/h
b. 10 mg/h
c. 15 mg/h
d. 20 mg/h
e. 30 mg/h

8. A 49-year-old male in end stage renal failure is able to perform peritoneal dialysis at home. The effective osmolarity (reflection coefficient) of the solution chosen for peritoneal dialysis will determine the rate of ultrafiltration. Which of the following statements best characterizes a molecule whose effective osmolarity (reflection coefficient) is zero?

a. It will not permeate the membrane
b. It can only cross the membrane through the lipid bilayer
c. It causes water to flow across the membrane
d. It is as diffusible through the membrane as water
e. It is transported across the membrane by a carrier

9. The characteristic of a water-insoluble substance most important in governing its diffusibility through a cell membrane is its

a. Hydrated diameter
b. Molecular weight
c. Electrical charge
d. Lipid solubility
e. Three-dimensional shape

10. Which one of the following muscle proteins plays an important role in contraction of both smooth and striated muscle?

a. Calmodulin
b. Troponin
c. Tropomyosin
d. Actin
e. Myosin light chains

11. A 32-year-old woman undergoing surgery for appendicitis develops malignant hyperthermia. Malignant hyperthermia is a life-threatening increase in metabolic rate that occasionally occurs when volatile anesthetics are used during surgery. It is caused by a mutation of the ryanodine receptor. Which one of the following best explains why a mutation of the ryanodine receptor can produce malignant hyperthermia?

a. A sustained release of calcium from the sarcoplasmic reticulum of skeletal muscle
b. Presynaptic terminals of alpha motoneurons undergo rapid repetitive firing
c. Skeletal muscle cells are unable to repolarize
d. A sudden cooling of the body causes uncontrollable shivering
e. Serum thyroxine levels increases to abnormally high levels

12. A 62-year-old male with COPD presents to the emergency room in respiratory distress. The attending physician uses succinylcholine to produce skeletal muscle relaxation prior to tracheal intubation. Soon after infusion of the succinylcholine the patient develops a severe bradycardia. Which one of the following drugs would counteract the bradycardia without affecting muscle relaxation?

a. Curare
b. Atropine
c. Epinephrine
d. Acetylcholine
e. Dopamine

13. Which one of the following conditions will produce a decrease in the magnitude of a nerve membrane action potential?

a. Decreasing the conductance of the membrane to potassium
b. Stimulating the nerve during the relative refractory period
c. Increasing the extracellular concentration of sodium
d. Making the membrane potential more negative
e. Increasing the magnitude of the stimulus

14. An 18-year-old male is brought to the emergency room by his friends after eating mushrooms. He is treated for muscarinic poisoning. Which one of the following signs is consistent with muscarinic poisoning?

a. Skeletal muscle contractures
b. Bradycardia
c. Dilation of the pupils
d. Hypertension
e. Diuresis

15. A 59-year-old male with an ejection fraction of 15%, who is being treated with medications for his heart failure, is asked whether he would like to participate in a trial for an experimental drug. The drug being tested is designed to decrease the expression of phospholamban on ventricular muscle cells. Which one of the following would be increased by decreasing phospholamban?

a. The activity of the sodium-potassium pump
b. The diastolic stiffness of the ventricular muscle cells
c. The activity of the L-type calcium channels
d. The duration of the ventricular muscle action potential
e. The concentration of calcium within the SR

16. A 35-year-old woman is seen by a neurologist to evaluate her incapacitating muscle weakness. The neurologist suspects myasthenia gravis and decides to confirm his diagnosis by administering a drug that increases the force of muscle contraction in patients with myasthenia gravis. Caution is advised when administering the drug to patients with heart disease because bradycardia may develop. Which one of the following most likely explains the ability of the drug to increase the force of muscle contraction in patients with myasthenia gravis?

a. Increasing the amount of acetylcholine released by alpha motoneurons
b. Increasing the affinity of the skeletal muscle acetylcholine receptors to acetylcholine
c. Increasing the alpha motoneuron discharge rate
d. Decreasing the metabolic breakdown rate of acetylcholine
e. Decreasing the concentration of calcium in the extracellular fluid

17. When comparing the contractile responses in smooth and skeletal muscle, which of the following is most different?

a. The source of activator calcium
b. The role of calcium in initiating contraction
c. The mechanism of force generation
d. The source of energy used during contraction
e. The nature of the contractile proteins

18. The amount of force produced by a skeletal muscle can be increased by

a. Increasing extracellular Mg^{2+}
b. Decreasing extracellular Ca^{2+}
c. Increasing the activity of acetylcholine esterase
d. Decreasing the interval between contractions
e. Increasing the preload beyond 2.2 μm

19. A 19-year-old woman with a history of diplopia and paresthesia is diagnosed with multiple sclerosis (MS). MS is a demyelinating disease characterized by a failure of nerve conduction. Immersion of an affected limb in a cold bath restores nerve conduction in many of these patients. The explanation often cited for this effect is that cold increases the duration of the action potential. Which one of the following best explains why increasing the duration of the action potential can restore nerve conduction in patients with MS?

a. The capacitance of the nerve fiber membrane is increased
b. The duration of the refractory period is increased
c. The potassium conductance of the membrane is increased
d. The amount of sodium entering the nerve with each action potential increases
e. The membrane potential becomes more positive

20. The rate of diffusion of a particle across a membrane will increase if

a. The area of the membrane decreases
b. The thickness of the membrane increases
c. The size of the particle increases
d. The concentration gradient of the particle decreases
e. The lipid solubility of the particle increases

21. A 32-year-old man sees his physician after collapsing suddenly without any other physical distress. Laboratory results demonstrate a higher-than-normal serum plasma concentration of potassium and he is diagnosed with periodic hyperkalemic paralysis, a clinical condition in which a sudden increase in extracellular potassium concentration results in muscle weakness. Which of the following is likely to cause muscle weakness as a result of increased extracellular potassium concentration?

a. Hyperpolarization of muscle cells
b. Inactivation of sodium channels in muscle cells
c. Increased release of neurotransmitters from alpha motoneurons
d. Decreased potassium conductance in muscle cells
e. Increased duration of action potentials produced by alpha motoneurons

22. The flow of calcium into the cell is an important component of the upstroke phase of action potentials in

a. Cardiac ventricular muscle
b. Intestinal smooth muscle
c. Skeletal muscle fibers
d. Nerve cell bodies
e. Presynaptic nerve terminals

23. The membrane potential will depolarize by the greatest amount if the membrane permeability increases for

a. Potassium
b. Sodium and potassium
c. Chloride
d. Potassium and chloride
e. Sodium

24. Which of the following will be less during the overshoot of an action potential than during the resting state?

a. Membrane conductance for sodium
b. Membrane conductance for potassium
c. Transference for sodium
d. Transference for potassium
e. Total membrane conductance

25. Preventing the inactivation of sodium channels will decrease

a. The relative refractory period of nerve cells
b. The upstroke velocity of nerve cell action potentials
c. The downstroke velocity of nerve cell action potentials
d. The magnitude of the overshoot in nerve cell action potentials
e. The duration of nerve cell action potentials

26. Connexin is an important component of the

a. Gap junction
b. Sarcoplasmic reticulum
c. Microtubule
d. Synaptic vesicle
e. Sodium channel

27. An increase in sodium conductance is associated with

a. The plateau phase of the ventricular muscle action potential
b. The downstroke of the skeletal muscle action potential
c. The upstroke of the smooth muscle action potential
d. The refractory period of the nerve cell action potential
e. The end-plate potential of the skeletal muscle fiber

28. Electrically excitable gates are normally involved in

a. The depolarization of the end-plate membrane by ACh
b. Hyperpolarization of the rods by light
c. Release of calcium from ventricular muscle SR
d. Transport of glucose into cells by a sodium-dependent, secondary active transport system
e. Increase in nerve cell potassium conductance caused by membrane depolarization

29. The sodium gradient across the nerve cell membrane is

a. A result of the Donnan equilibrium
b. Significantly changed during an action potential
c. Used as a source of energy for the transport of other ions
d. An important determinant of the resting membrane potential
e. Maintained by a Na^+/Ca^{2+} exchanger

30. A 16-year-old boy on the track team asks his pediatrician if he can take creatine on a regular basis in order to increase his muscle strength prior to a track meet. He wants to take creatine because

a. Creatine increases plasma glucose concentration
b. Creatine prevents dehydration
c. Creatine increases muscle glycogen concentrations
d. Creatine is converted to phosphocreatine
e. Creatine delays the metabolism of fatty acids

31. Which of the following would cause an immediate reduction in the amount of potassium leaking out of a cell?

a. Increasing the permeability of the membrane to potassium
b. Increasing (hyperpolarizing) the membrane potential
c. Decreasing the extracellular potassium concentration
d. Reducing the activity of the sodium-potassium pump
e. Decreasing the extracellular sodium concentration

32. A 32-year-old male is diagnosed with primary hypertension. His physician recommends a new drug for hypertension that acts by decreasing vascular smooth-muscle contractile activity without affecting ventricular contractility. The most likely site of action for the new drug is

a. Beta receptors
b. Calmodulin
c. Troponin
d. Tropomyosin
e. Protein kinase A

33. Synaptic transmission between pain fibers from the skin and spinal cord neurons is mediated by

a. Acetylcholine
b. Substance P
c. Endorphins
d. Somatostatin
e. Serotonin

34. Which one of the following transport processes is a passive downhill process?

a. Sodium out of brain cells
b. Calcium into the SR
c. Hydrogen into the lumen of canaliculi of the parietal cells of the stomach
d. Glucose into the fat cells of adipose tissue
e. Phosphate into epithelial cells lining the proximal tubule of the kidney

Questions 35–36

Use the following diagram to answer the questions.

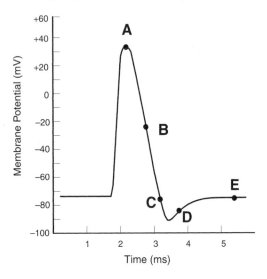

35. At which point on the action potential does the Na^+ current exceed the K^+ current?

a. Point A
b. Point B
c. Point C
d. Point D
e. Point E

36. At which point on the action potential is the membrane closest to the Na^+ equilibrium potential?

a. Point A
b. Point B
c. Point C
d. Point D
e. Point E

37. A 64-year-old male was admitted to the hospital with edema and congestive heart failure. He was found to have diastolic dysfunction characterized by inadequate filling of the heart during diastole. The decrease in ventricular filling is due to a decrease in ventricular muscle compliance. Which one of the following proteins determines the normal stiffness of ventricular muscle?

a. Calmodulin
b. Troponin
c. Tropomyosin
d. Titin
e. Myosin light chain kinase

38. The activity of the calcium pump on the SR of cardiac muscle is regulated by

a. Inositol triphosphate
b. Myosin light chain kinase
c. Phospholamban
d. Protein kinase A
e. Phospholipase C

39. A 16-year-old, highly allergic girl who is stung by a bee gives herself a shot of epinephrine using a syringe and needle prescribed by her physician. Because epinephrine activities beta-receptors, it will relieve the effects of the bee sting by decreasing

a. The contraction of airway smooth muscle
b. The strength of ventricular muscle contraction
c. The rate of depolarization in the SA node
d. The transport of calcium into skeletal muscle fibers
e. The rate of glycogenolysis in the liver

40. A 61-year-old male with erectile disfunction asks his physician to prescribe Viagra (sildenafil). Viagra produces its physiological effects by blocking the enzyme that hydrolyzes the second messenger by which nitric oxide produces its physiological effects. The second messenger is

a. Bradykinin
b. Cyclic GMP
c. Protein kinase A
d. Endothelin
e. Inositol triphosphate

41. The NMDA receptor is activated by

a. Glycine
b. Acetylcholine
c. Substance P
d. Histamine
e. Glutamate

Questions 42–43

Use the following diagram, which illustrates the chemical reactions that occur during cross-bridge cycling in smooth muscle, to answer the following two questions.

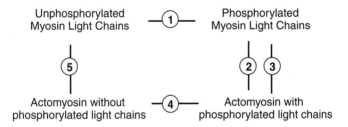

42. Which one of the following enzymes is responsible for step 1 in the diagram?

a. Calmodulin
b. Protein kinase A
c. Myosin light chain kinase
d. Phospholipase C
e. Actomyosin ATPase

43. Which one of the steps in the diagram is responsible for the formation of latch bridges?

a. Step 1
b. Step 2
c. Step 3
d. Step 4
e. Step 5

44. A 42-year-old woman is seen in consultation by a dermatologist to evaluate and treat her glabellar lines (frown lines on the forehead just above the nose). After her treatment options are explained, the patient asks the dermatologist to administer Botox (botulinum type A). Botox injections smooth out the lines on the forehead by

a. Blocking the release of synaptic transmitter from alpha motoneurons
b. Preventing the opening of sodium channels on muscle membranes
c. Decreasing the amount of calcium releases from the SR
d. Increasing the flow of blood into the facial muscle
e. Enhancing the enzymatic hydrolysis of acetylcholine at the neuromuscular junction

Cellular Physiology

Answers

1. The answer is c. (*Guyton, pp 62–65. Boron pp 289–290.*) The conduction velocity of an action potential along an axon is proportional to the axon's diameter for both unmyelinated and myelinated axons. The resting membrane potential, the duration of the relative refractory period, and the magnitude of the action potential are dependent on the type and density of electrically excitable gates and the ability of the Na^+,K^+-ATPase to establish and maintain the concentration gradients. These characteristics are not related in any systematic way to the axon diameter.

2. The answer is e. (*Guyton, p 714. Boron pp 406–411.*) Rapid removal of fluid from the brain can be produced by the administration of a fluid that increases the osmotic pressure difference between the brain and the cerebral vessels. The appropriate solution must have a higher-than-normal osmolarity (that is, greater than 300 mM) and be composed of a solute that is impermeable to the blood-brain barrier. Of the solutions listed, only urea and mannitol are hyperosmotic and of these, only mannitol is impermeable to the blood-brain barrier.

3. The answer is c. (*Guyton, pp 52–55. Boron, pp 814–817.*) Orange juice contains a significant amount of K^+. Consuming a large amount of K^+ when the extracellular volume is low (dehydration) can cause a significant rise in extracellular K^+. An increase in extracellular K^+ makes the membrane potential more positive. Depolarizing the membrane opens K^+ channels causing an increace in membrane conductance. Prolonged depolarization, whether caused by an increase in extracellular K^+ or by an action potential causes Na^+ channels to inactivate. Inactivation, which decreases the excitability of the nerve membrane, is observed in hyperkalemia and during the absolute and relative refractory periods following a normal action potential. The activity of the Na-K pump can be reduced by a reduction, not an increase, in extracellular K^+ concentration.

4. The answer is d. (*Boron, pp 61–63.*) Digoxin is used to treat atrial fibrillation because it increases vagal tone and to treat congestive heart failure because it increases cardiac contractility. Digoxin produces its physiological effects by blocking the K^+ binding site on the Na-K pump. When the extracellular K^+ concentration is low, digoxin produces a greater than expected inhibition of the Na-K pump.

5. The answer is b. *(Boron, pp 181–183. Guyton, p 59.)* Membrane excitability is related to the ease with which depolarization opens Na^+ channels. The opening of the Na^+ channel in response to depolarization is, in part, related to the extracellular Ca^{2+} concentration; the lower the extracellular Ca^{2+} concentration, the easier it is for Na^+ channels to open when the membrane depolarizes. Hyperventilation (lowering arterial CO_2 tension) decreases extracellular Ca^{2+} concentration by increasing arterial pH. When pH rises, H^+ is released from plasma proteins in exchange for Ca^{2+}, and ionized Ca^{2+} concentration decreases.

6. The answer is a. *(Boron, pp 815–817. Guyton, pp 106, 132–133.)* Hyperkalemia is a life-threatening emergency that can be recognized by the peaked T waves observed on an electrocardiogram. The peaked T waves are produced by an accelerated repolarization of ventricular muscle. Potentially fatal hyperkalemia is treated by administering insulin (along with glucose), which helps K^+ transport into cells and therefore lowers extracellular K^+.

7. The answer is e. *(Guyton, pp 40–45. Boron, pp 54–56.)* Fick's law states that diffusional flux is proportional to the concentration difference (Flux $\propto$ [$C_1 - C_2$]). Doubling the concentration of the substance in chamber A causes the concentration difference to increase by threefold. Therefore, the flux increases from 10 to 30 mg/h.

8. The answer is d. *(Guyton, pp 45–47, 269–271, 378. Boron, pp 77–78.)* The reflection coefficient is a measure of a membrane's permeability to a substance in comparison to its permeability to water. It can be calculated from the following equation:

$$\text{Reflection coefficient} = [P(\text{water}) - P(\text{substance})]/P(\text{water})$$

It is also a measure of the actual osmotic pressure developed by the substance compared with the osmotic pressure that it should theoretically develop according to van't Hoff's equation. A substance with a reflection coefficient of zero would have the same diffusibility through the membrane as water and would not develop any osmotic pressure.

9. The answer is d. (*Guyton, pp 40–42. Boron, pp 54–56.*) Materials that are not soluble in water can only cross the membrane through the lipid bilayer. The most important factor determining how well a substance can diffuse across the lipid bilayer is the substance's lipid solubility. If two materials have the same lipid solubility, then the permeability of the smaller particle will be greater.

10. The answer is d. (*Guyton, pp 71, 84–86, 89–90. Boron, pp 240–245.*) In both smooth and striated muscle, contraction is produced by the cross-bridge cycle in which the cross-bridge on the thick filament binds to the actin molecule on the thin filament. In excitation-contraction coupling in striated muscle, calcium initiates contraction by binding to troponin. The calcium-activated troponin then acts to remove the tropomyosin-mediated inhibition of the actin-myosin interaction. In excitation-contraction coupling in smooth muscle, calcium initiates contraction by binding to calmodulin. The calcium-activated calmodulin then activates the myosin light chain protein kinase (MLCK) enzyme, which phosphorylates the myosin light chains. Actin-myosin interaction follows light-chain phosphorylation.

11. The answer is a. (*Guyton, pp 84–86. Boron, pp 241–243.*) The ryanodine receptor or calcium release channel on the sarcoplasmic reticulum (SR) is normally opened when skeletal muscle is activated. The flow of calcium through the open ryanodine receptor binds to troponin and initiates muscle contraction. The metabolic activity accompanying muscle contraction can warm the body. If a mutation in the ryanodine receptor causes uncontrolled release of calcium from the SR, the body temperature can rise to levels that cause brain damage.

12. The answer is b. (*Guyton, pp 80–83. Boron, pp 209–213.*) Succinylcholine is a rapidly active neuromuscular blocking agent with a very short duration. Respiratory paralysis can be produced in less than 60 seconds and normal respiration typically returns within 15 minutes. Because succinylcholine can also stimulate autonomic postganglionic fibers, vagal fibers innervating the heart are stimulated. The vagal fibers release acetylcholine choline which binds to muscarinic receptors on the SA node, slowing the heart. The bradycardia can be prevented by administering atropine, which blocks the muscarinic receptors on the SA node.

13. The answer is b. (*Guyton, pp 55–59. Boron, pp 176–178.*) An action potential is normally an all-or-none response; that is, its magnitude is independent of the stimulus strength. The magnitude of the action potential is reduced during the relative refractory period or when the membrane is depolarized by an abnormally high extracellular potassium concentration. The upstroke of the action potential is caused by an inward flow of sodium ions, and therefore its magnitude depends on the extracellular sodium concentration.

14. The answer is b. (*Guyton, pp 700–703. Boron, pp 386–389.*) Muscarine binds to acetylcholine muscarinic receptors on cardiac and smooth muscle. These are the same receptors activated by the release of acetylcholine by the vagus nerve. Cardiac muscarinic receptors slow phase 4 depolarization and therefore, the heart rate. A heart rate less than 60 beats per minute is called bradycardia. Acetylcholine receptors on the skeletal muscle end plate are nicotinic receptors and do not respond to muscarine. Dilation of the pupils and hypertension are signs of sympathetic, not parasympathetic activity.

15. The answer is e. (*Guyton, pp 98–99. Boron, pp 244–245, 524–557.*) Phospholamban is a protein contained within the SR that inhibits the activity of the SR calcium pump. Inactivation of phospholamban results in an increase in calcium sequestration by the SR. Increasing the concentration of calcium within the SR increases the force of the ventricular contraction.

16. The answer is d. (*Guyton, p 83. Boron, pp 224, 227–229.*) The drug used to test for myasthenia gravis is an acetylcholinesterase inhibitor such as neostigmine. The drug prevents the breakdown of acetylcholine, increasing the duration of time acetylcholine remains in the synaptic cleft. Because acetylcholine can bind to the end-plate receptors for a longer time, the magnitude of the end-plate potential increases, increasing the probability of it generating an action potential. The greater the action potential force rate, the greater the source of muscle contraction. Increasing the amount of acetylcholine released by the alpha motoneurons, by increasing the affinity of the skeletal muscle receptors for acetylcholine or increasing the discharge rate of alpha motoneurons could cause a similar effect. However, none of these changes would affect heart rate. The cautious use of this test in patients with heart failure results from the possibility that the decreased breakdown of acetylcholine released by the vagus nerve could decrease heart rate to dangerously low levels.

17. The answer is b. (*Guyton, pp 84–86, 89–90. Boron, 236–238.*) The greatest difference in excitation-contraction coupling involves the role of calcium in initiating contraction. In smooth muscle, calcium binds to and activates calmodulin, which, by activating myosin light chain kinase (MLCK), catalyzes the phosphorylation of the 20,000-Da myosin light chain (LC_{20}). Once the light chains are phosphorylated, myosin cross-bridges bind to actin on the thin filaments, which initiates contraction. In skeletal muscle, calcium binds to troponin, which removes the tropomyosin-mediated inhibition of the actin-myosin interactions. Once the inhibition is removed, cross-bridge cycling (and contraction) begins. In both smooth and skeletal muscle, the cycling of cross-bridges generates force. ATP provides the energy for the cycling of the cross-bridges in both muscles. In skeletal muscle, activator calcium comes exclusively from the SR, whereas in smooth muscle calcium can come from both the SR and the extracellular fluid.

18. The answer is d. (*Guyton, p 76. Boron, pp 249–250.*) When the interval between skeletal muscle contractions is small, the force produced by the two successive contractions will summate. The shorter the interval between the contractions, the greater the summation will be. Maximum summation is called tetanus. Decreasing extracellular Ca^{2+} will increase the excitability of skeletal muscle fibers but does not have a direct effect on contractile force. Increasing the Mg^{2+} concentration will decrease skeletal muscle excitability. Increasing the preload beyond 2.2 μm decreases the overlap between thick and thin filaments and therefore decreases the force of contraction. Increasing the activity of acetylcholine esterase enhances the hydrolysis of ACh and therefore decreases the likelihood that muscle contraction will be initiated.

19. The answer is d. (*Guyton, pp 59–60, 62–63. Boron, pp 292–293.*) In order for propagation of an action potential to occur, the depolarization produced by one action potential must depolarize the adjacent patch of excitable membrane to threshold. In demyelinating diseases, such as multiple sclerosis, too much charge leaks from the membrane and as a result, not enough is available to bring the next patch of membrane to threshold. Increasing the duration of the action potential increases the amount of charge entering the cell and therefore increases the probability that the next patch of excitable membrane will be depolarized to threshold. Increasing the duration of the refractory period will not affect the amount of charge entering the cell. Depolarizing the membrane and increasing potassium conductance will make it more difficult to produce an action potential. If membrane capacitance is increased, the amount of charge required to excite the next patch of membrane will be increased.

20. The answer is e. *(Guyton, pp 40–42. Boron, p 56.)* The rate of diffusion is described by Fick's law, which states that the flux of material across a membrane is directly proportional to the area of a membrane and the concentration difference of the particles on either side of the membrane and is inversely proportional to the thickness of the membrane. In general, if all other properties of the membrane are the same, the greater the lipid solubility of a particle, the greater its concentration in the membrane and, therefore, the greater its flux across the membrane.

21. The answer is b. *(Guyton, pp 56–57, 64. Boron, pp 149–150, 188–189.)* Periodic hyperkalemic paralysis is caused by inactivation of the skeletal muscle membranes. Inactivation is produced by depolarization of the skeletal muscle membrane, which occurs when extracellular potassium concentration increases. Inactivation of the sodium channels on the skeletal muscle membrane prevents action potentials from being produced and therefore leads to muscle weakness or paralysis. Although the exact mechanism of periodic hyperkalemic paralysis is not known, it appears to be due to a mutation in the gene coding for the sodium inactivation gate.

22. The answer is b. *(Guyton, pp 56–59, 91–92, 97–98. Boron, pp 176–177, 232, 486–487.)* In intestinal smooth muscle, the upstroke of the action potential is caused by the flow of calcium into the cell. In cells of the cardiac ventricular muscle, the plateau phase of the action potential, but not the upstroke, is accompanied by the flow of calcium into the cells. Skeletal muscle fibers resemble nerve fibers. In both of these cells, the upstroke of the action potential is caused by the flow of sodium into the cell.

23. The answer is e. (*Guyton, pp 52–55, 521–523. Boron, pp 153–154, 306–308.*) When the permeability of a particular ion is increased, the membrane potential moves toward the equilibrium potential for that ion. The equilibrium potentials for chloride (−80 mV) and potassium (−92 mV) are close to the resting membrane potential, so increases in their permeability have little effect on the resting membrane potential. The equilibrium potential for sodium (+60 mV) is very far from the resting membrane potential. Thus, increasing the permeability for sodium causes a large depolarization.

24. The answer is d. (*Guyton, pp 55–56, 58–59. Boron, pp 154–156, 176–178.*) During an action potential, the conductance for both sodium and potassium is higher than it is at rest. However, the conductance for sodium is higher than the conductance for potassium during the overshoot. Hence, the transference for potassium is less. Recall that transference is a measure of an ion's relative conductance:

$$T_{Na} = g_{Na}/(g_{Na} + g_K) \quad \text{and} \quad T_K = g_K/(g_{Na} + g_K)$$

where T = transference and g = conductance.

25. The answer is c. (*Guyton, p 64. Boron, pp 181–182.*) The repolarization phase of the action potential is produced by a decrease in Na^+ conductance, due to the inactivation of Na^+ channels, and the increase in K^+ conductance, due to the activation of K^+ channels. Preventing the inactivation of Na^+ channels will decrease the downstroke velocity of the action potential. This will slow the normal repolarization phase of the action potential and thereby prolong the duration of the action potential. The relative refractory period is prolonged because of the prolonged duration of the action potential. The upstroke velocity and the magnitude depend on how rapidly and how long the sodium channels are opened. By preventing inactivation of the Na^+ channel, the rate of the upstroke and the magnitude of the overshoot may be increased.

26. The answer is a. (*Guyton, p 515. Boron, pp 164–165.*) Connexin is a membrane-spanning protein that is used to create gap junction channels. The gap junction channel creates a cytoplasmic passage between two cells. Each cell membrane contains half of the channel. The channel, called a connexon, is constructed from six connexin molecules that form a cylinder with a pore at its center.

27. The answer is e. (*Guyton, pp 80–82. Boron, pp 209–213.*) The channel opened by ACh when it binds to receptors on the end plates of skeletal muscle fibers is equally permeable to potassium and sodium. The increase in sodium permeability allows sodium to flow into the cell and produces the end-plate potential. The plateau phase of ventricular muscle action potentials and the upstroke of smooth muscle action potentials are produced by an increase in calcium conductance. An increase in potassium conductance is responsible for the downstroke of the action potential. The refractory period is caused by an increase in potassium conductance and a decrease in the number of sodium channels available to produce an action potential (i.e., sodium channel inactivation).

28. The answer is e. (*Guyton, pp 56–58. Boron, pp 193–194, 814–816.*) Electrically excitable gates are those that respond to a change in membrane potential. The most notable electrically excitable gates are those on the sodium and potassium channels that produce the nerve action potential. The potassium channel gate is opened by depolarization. Ventricular muscle SR releases its calcium in response to an increase in intracellular calcium. The gates opened by ACh are chemically excitable gates. In rods, sodium channels are closed when cGMP is hydrolyzed. Electrically excitable gates do not regulate the active transport of glucose.

29. The answer is c. (*Guyton, pp 47–50. Boron, pp 66–69.*) The sodium-potassium pump uses the energy contained in ATP to maintain the sodium gradient across the membrane. The sodium gradient, in turn, is used to transport other substances across the membrane. For example, the Na/Ca exchanger uses the energy in the sodium gradient to help maintain the low intracellular calcium required for normal cell function. Although sodium enters the cell during an action potential, the quantity of sodium is so small that no significant change in intracellular sodium concentration occurs. Because the sodium transference is so low, the sodium equilibrium potential is not an important determinant of the resting membrane potential.

30. The answer is d. (*Guyton, pp 74, 816, 968–970. Boron, pp 1244–1245.*) Phosphocreatine is rapidly converted to ATP in muscle. When the metabolic demands exceed the rate at which ATP can be generated by aerobic metabolism or glycolysis, phosphocreatine can supply the necessary ATP for a brief period of time. An increase in the concentration of phosphocreatine in muscle may increase the amount of ATP that can be produced and therefore enhance performance.

31. The answer is b. (*Guyton, pp 54–55. Boron, pp 156–157.*) The amount of potassium leaking out of the cell depends on its driving forces and its membrane conductance. The driving forces are the membrane potential and the concentration gradient. Hyperpolarizing the membrane makes the inside of the cell more negative and therefore, makes it more difficult for potassium to flow out of the cell. Increasing the permeability of the membrane to potassium or decreasing the extracellular potassium concentration increases the flow of potassium out of the cell. Altering the activity of the sodium-potassium pump or the extracellular sodium concentration has no immediate effect on the flow of potassium across the membrane. However, decreasing the activity of the sodium-potassium pump will ultimately depolarize the membrane, increasing the flow of potassium out of the cell.

32. The answer is b. (*Guyton, p 90. Boron, pp 236–238.*) Smooth muscle contraction is regulated by a series of reactions that begins with the binding of calcium to calmodulin. The calcium-calmodulin complex then binds to and activates a protein kinase called myosin light chain kinase (MLCK). MLCK catalyzes the phosphorylation of the myosin light chains (LC_{20}). Once these light chains are phosphorylated, myosin and actin interaction can occur and the muscle shortens and develops tension. Calcium initiates contraction in striated muscle by binding to troponin, which by altering the position of tropomyosin on the thin filament, allows cross-bridge cycling to begin. Although beta receptor agonists may lower blood pressure by relaxing vascular smooth muscle, they also increase the rate and strength of the heart beat.

33. The answer is b. (*Guyton, pp 552–555. Boron, pp 356–357.*) Substance P is an 11-amino acid polypeptide found in neurons within the hypothalamus and spinal cord. It is released from small A delta and C fibers that relay information from nociceptors to neurons within the substantia gelatinosa of the spinal cord. Endorphins and other opioid neurotransmitters may partially inhibit the perception of pain by presynaptically inhibiting the release of substance P from nociceptor afferent fibers.

34. The answer is d. *(Guyton, pp 742–743, 885–886. Boron, pp 894–895, 1078–1081.)* Glucose is transported into fat cells by facilitated diffusion and thus does not require the direct or indirect use of energy. Insulin increases the rate of diffusion but is not necessary for the diffusion. All of the other transport systems require energy. Sodium is transported out of cells by Na-K ATPase; calcium is transported into the SR by a Ca ATPase; and hydrogen is transported from the parietal cells of the stomach by a H-K ATPase. All of these transporters use ATP directly in the transport process. In the proximal tubule, phospate is transported into the luminal cells of the proximal tubule by a $Na-HPO_4$ secondary active transport system.

35–36. The answers are 35-d, 36-a. *(Guyton, pp 55–59. Boron, pp 164–165, 176–177.)* When the inward Na current exceeds the outward potassium current, the membrane potential depolarizes toward the Na^+ equilibrium potential. The only point on the diagram in which the membrane is depolarizing is point **D**. When the K^+ current exceeds the Na^+ current, the membrane potential hyperpolarizes toward the K^+ equilibrium potential. When the membrane potential is not changing, for example, at points **A** and **E**, the two currents are equal.

The Na^+ equilibrium potential is usually between +60 and +70 mV, depending on the ratio of the intracellular and extracellular Na^+ concentrations. During an action potential, the peak of the action potential (point **A**) is close, but not equal, to the Na^+ equilibrium potential. The membrane potential doesn't reach the Na^+ equilibrium potential because the Na^+ channels start to inactivate and the K^+ channels begin to activate during the upstroke of the action potential.

37. The answer is d. *(Guyton, pp 72–73. Boron, pp 235, 525–527.)* Titin is a large protein that located between the Z line at the end of the sarcomere to the M line in the middle of the sarcomere. The resistance of the muscle to stretch is determined by the elasticity of the titin molecule. The titin in cardiac muscle is much stiffer than in the skeletal muscle, so it is more difficult to stretch cardiac muscle cells than it is to stretch skeletal muscle fibers.

38. The answer is c. (Boron, pp 245–246, 523.) Phospholamban regulates the activity of the SR calcium pump in cardiac muscle. The inhibition is reduced when phospholamban is phosphorylated by a cAMP-dependent kinase called protein kinase A. When the ventricular muscle beta receptors are activated by sympathetic stimulation or circulating catecholamines, they activate a G protein, which, in turn, activates adenylyl cyclase. Adenylyl cyclase catalyzes the formation of cAMP, which activates protein kinase A.

39. The answer is a. (Boron, p 626. Guyton, p 440.) Beta-receptor-activated G proteins activate adenyl cyclase, which catalyzes the formation of cAMP. cAMP activates protein kinase A, which phosphorylates phospholamban. Phosphorylated phospholamban releases the SR Ca^{2+} pump from inhibition. The sequestration of Ca^{2+} into the SR relaxes bronchiolar smooth muscle. In cardiac muscle, the sequestration of Ca^{2+} into the SR increases contractile strength because there is more Ca^{2+} available for release with each action potential. The depolarization of the SA node is caused by activation of the "funny" channel. This channel is activated at negative membrane potentials. The rate of its activation is increased when it is phosphorylated by protein kinase A. The transport of Ca^{2+} into skeletal muscle fibers is not affected by beta receptors. Glycogenolysis in the liver is also increased by activated beta receptors. In this case, the protein kinase A phosphorylates an enzyme called phosphorylase, which begins the process of glycogenolysis.

40. The answer is b. (Guyton, pp 93, 520, 921. Boron, pp 108–110, 1136–1139.) Viagra (sildenafil) is an effective and selective inhibitor of cGMP phosphodiseterase. Erections are produced by the release of NO, which inhibits the smooth muscle of the corpus caverosa, allowing blood to fill the penis. NO increases the synthesis of cGMP, which produces smooth muscle relaxation. By blocking the breakdown of cGMP, Viagra prolongs the action of NO and erections.

41. The answer is e. (Boron, pp 313–316.) The NMDA receptor channel is a large channel permeable to Ca^{2+}, K^+, and Na^+. It is activated by glutamate, but unlike other glutamate receptor channels, the NMDA channel is blocked by Mg^{2+} in its resting state. Depolarization of the cell membrane to approximately −40 mV removes the Mg^{2+} blockade. Therefore, the NMDA channel is only opened when the cell is depolarized by other excitatory neurotransmitters. The Ca^{2+} entering the cell activates a number of intracellular enzymes, some of which may be involved in memory.

42–43. The answers are 42-c, 43-d. (*Boron, pp 237–238, 244–245, 250–251. Guyton, pp 89–90.*) Cross-bridge cycling in smooth muscle cannot begin until the myosin light chains are phosphorylated (step 1). Phosphorylation is enzymatically stimulated by myosin light chain kinase (MLCK). Phospholipase C is a phosphodiesterase enzyme that catalyzes the hydrolysis of PIP_2 to IP_3. IP_3 promotes the release of Ca^{2+} from the SR. Ca^{2+} activates calmodulin, which, in turn, activates MLCK. Latch bridges are unphosphorylated myosin cross-bridges that are bound to actin. These cross-bridges cycle very slowly or not at all and are responsible for the ability of smooth muscle to maintain its tone for a long time without expending energy for cross-bridge cycling. The enzyme myosin light chain phosphatase is responsible for dephosphorylating cycling cross-bridges. The smooth muscle relaxes when Ca^{2+} is removed from the myoplasm and the latch bridges detach from actin.

44. The answer is a. (*Boron, pp 226–227. Guyton, pp 82–83.*) Botulinum toxin inhibits the release of acetylcholine from alpha motoneurons by blocking one of the proteins responsible for the fusion of the synaptic channel with the presynaptic membrane. Botulinum toxin also inhibits the release of acetylcholine from the neurons of the autonomic nervous system. Botulinum and tetanus toxin are released from the same class of bacteria (*Clostridium*). Tetanus toxin produces an increase in skeletal muscle contraction by blocking the release of inhibitory neurotransmitter from spinal interneurons.

Cardiac Physiology

Questions

DIRECTIONS: Each question below contains five suggested responses. Select the **one best** response to each question.

45. A 32-year-old male was admitted to the hospital with an initial diagnosis of heart failure. Cardiac catheterization was performed to measure cardiac output using the Fick principle. Use the following data to calculate the cardiac output. Pulmonary artery O_2 content = 20 ml/100 ml; Pulmonary vein O_2 content = 12 ml/100 ml; oxygen consumption = 280 ml/min.

a. 2.5 L/min
b. 3.5 L/min
c. 4.5 L/min
d. 6.0 L/min
e. 8.0 L/min

46. A 42-year-old woman with mitral prolapse is admitted to the hospital for evaluation of her cardiac function. Which of the following values is the best index of the preload on her heart?

a. Blood volume
b. Central venous pressure
c. Pulmonary capillary wedge pressure
d. Left ventricular end-diastolic volume
e. Left ventricular end-diastolic pressure

47. A patient presents to the emergency room with intermittent chest pain. The EKG and blood tests are negative for an MI (myocardial infarction). However an echocardiogram shows some thickening of the left ventricular muscle and narrowing of the aortic valve. Medications to lower afterload are prescribed. Which of the following values should be measured to determine if the medications have been effective in lowering left ventricular afterload?

a. Left ventricular end-diastolic pressure
b. Left ventricular mean systolic pressure
c. Pulmonary capillary wedge pressure
d. Total peripheral resistance
e. Mean arterial blood pressure

48. The highest blood flow per gram of left ventricular myocardium would occur

a. When aortic pressure is highest
b. When left ventricular pressure is highest
c. At the beginning of isovolumic contraction
d. When aortic blood flow is highest
e. At the beginning of diastole

49. A 55-year-old male presents to the emergency room with a history of syncope. Which of the following cardiac conditions is most likely to have caused the patient's syncope?

a. Sinus arrhythmia
b. First-degree heart block
c. Second-degree heart block
d. Third-degree heart block
e. Tachycardia

50. During a routine physical examination, a 32-year-old female is found to have second-degree heart block. Which of the following ECG recordings was obtained from the patient during her physical examination?

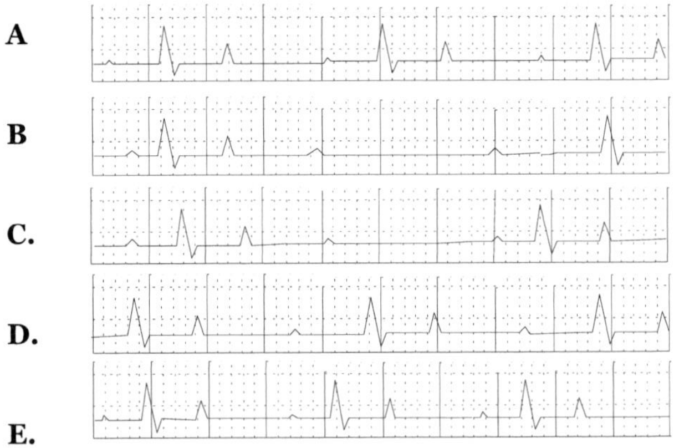

a. A
b. B
c. C
d. D
e. E

51. The following 6-lead frontal ECG was perfumed as part of an annual physical exam. What is the MEA (mean electrical axis) of the patient?

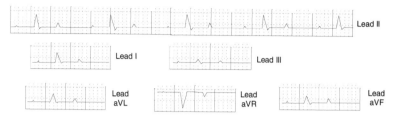

a. −10 degrees
b. +10 degrees
c. +20 degrees
d. +40 degrees
e. +70 degrees

52. During ventricular ejection, the pressure difference smallest in magnitude is between the

a. Pulmonary artery and left atrium
b. Right ventricle and right atrium
c. Left ventricle and aorta
d. Left ventricle and left atrium
e. Aorta and capillaries

53. An echocardiogram is performed on a 66-year-old male to assess ejection fraction and ventricular hypertrophy in a patient diagnosed with aortic regurgitation following a physical examination. Which of the following signs would be present in a patient with aortic regurgitation?

a. A decrease in diastolic pressure
b. A decrease in pulse pressure
c. A systolic murmur
d. A decrease in heart rate
e. A decrease in heart size

54. Stroke volume is increased by which of the following?

a. A decrease in venous compliance
b. An increase in afterload
c. A decrease in contractility
d. An increase in heart rate
e. A decrease in coronary blood flow

55. An increased preload would most likely be caused by which of the following?

a. An increase in TPR
b. A decrease in blood volume
c. An increase in myocardial contractility
d. A decrease in heart rate
e. An increase in venous capacitance

56. Propagation of the action potential through the heart is fastest in the

a. SA node
b. Atrial muscle
c. AV node
d. Purkinje fibers
e. Ventricular muscle

57. A 75-year-old woman with fatigue and shortness of breath improves markedly after the administration of a drug that increases the inotropic state of her heart. Which of the following changes is primarily responsible for the improvement in her condition?

a. A reduction in heart rate
b. A reduction in heart size
c. An increase in end-diastolic pressure
d. An increase in wall thickness
e. An increase in cardiac excitability

Questions 58–59

Use the pressure-volume curve illustrated below to determine the ejection fraction and diastolic pressure.

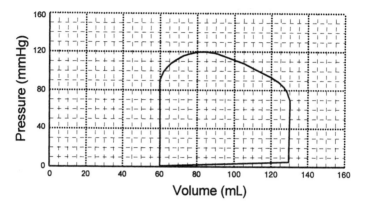

58. The ejection fraction equals

a. 0.50
b. 0.55
c. 0.60
d. 0.65
e. 0.70

59. The diastolic pressure equals

a. 0 mmHg
b. 5 mmHg
c. 70 mmHg
d. 90 mmHg
e. 120 mmHg

60. Closure of the aortic valve occurs at the onset of which phase of the cardiac cycle?

a. Isovolumetric contraction
b. Rapid ejection
c. Systole
d. Isovolumetric relaxation
e. Rapid filling

61. If the QRS complex is positive in leads II and a VF and a negative in lead III, the mean electrical axis (MEA) is between

a. −30° and 0°
b. 0° and +30°
c. +30° and +60°
d. +60° and +90°
e. +90° and +120°

62. An ECG obtained from a 57-year-old male during a routine physical examination reveals atrial fibrillation. Which of the following is most likely to accompany this condition?

a. An increased venous A wave
b. An increased left atrial pressure
c. A decreased heart rate
d. An increased stroke volume
e. An increased arterial blood pressure

63. Normal splitting of the second heart sound (S_2) into two components is increased during inspiration because

a. The closing of the aortic valve is delayed
b. The opening of the mitral valve is delayed
c. The closing of the pulmonic valve is delayed
d. The stroke volume of the left ventricle is increased
e. The heart rate is decreased

64. During a routine examination of a 55-year-old female, a third heart sound (S_3) is heard. Which of the following conditions most likely caused the third heart sound to be heard?

a. Right bundle branch block
b. Left heart failure
c. Mitral stenosis
d. Aortic regurgitation
e. Tachycardia

65. A 23-year-old female presents with fatigue and is found to have a higher-than-normal cardiac output. Which of the following conditions most likely produced her fatigue?

a. Hypertension
b. Aortic regurgitation
c. Anemia
d. Third-degree heart block
e. Cardiac tamponade

66. The diagram below illustrates the pressure-volume curves for two different hearts. Which of the following is greater in curve 1?

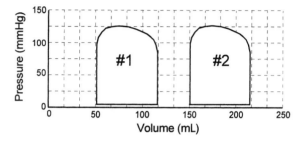

a. Preload
b. Work
c. Energy consumption
d. Efficiency
e. Stroke volume

67. A diagnostic evaluation of a 41-year-old male reveals a systolic murmur. The physician also notes a 7-cm distance between the height of the blood in his right internal jugular vein and sternal angle (normal = 3 cm). Which of the following conditions is most likely responsible for the physical findings?

a. Mitral stenosis
b. Tricuspid regurgitation
c. Atherosclerosis
d. Aortic regurgitation
e. Tachycardia

68. A 42-year-old woman with lightheadedness and recurrent syncope is rushed to the emergency room where she is given atropine. Her symptoms are relieved by an increase in which of the following?

a. Heart rate
b. PR interval
c. Ventricular contractility
d. Ejection fraction
e. Stroke volume

69. During exercise, there is an increase in a person's

a. Stroke volume
b. Diastolic pressure
c. Venous compliance
d. Pulmonary arterial resistance
e. Total peripheral resistance

70. Phase-4 depolarization of SA nodal cells is caused by which of the following?

a. An increase in the flow of sodium into the cell
b. A decrease in the flow of potassium out of the cell
c. An increase in the activity of the Na/Ca exchanger
d. A decrease in the flow of chloride out of the cell
e. A decrease in the activity of the Na-K pump

71. A patient seen by his doctor complains of fatigue and labored breathing. During auscultation of the heart, the physician notes that the splitting of the second heart sound is reversed: P2 occurs before A2. This paradoxical splitting of the second heart sound is most likely caused by which of the following?

a. An increase in right ventricular preload
b. A decrease in left ventricular contractility
c. An increase in systemic blood pressure
d. A decrease in heart rate
e. An increase in pulmonary vascular resistance

72. Blood pressure increases and heart rate decreases in response to which of the following?

a. Exercise
b. Increased body temperature
c. Exposure to high altitude
d. Increased intracranial pressure
e. Hemorrhage

73. During exercise, cardiac output is augmented by

a. Sympathetic stimulation of resistance vessels
b. Dilation of venous vessels
c. Decreased end-diastolic volume
d. Decreased mean systemic arterial pressure
e. Increased ventricular contractility

74. A 45-year-old woman makes an appointment to see her physician because she is having breathing difficulties when she lies down at night. An S_3 gallop is heard upon auscultation. Her signs and symptoms are most likely due to

a. Hypertension
b. Mitral regurgitation
c. Cor pulmonale
d. Cardiac pericarditis
e. Left heart failure

75. Stroke volume can be decreased by which of the following?

a. Increasing ventricular contractility
b. Increasing heart rate
c. Increasing central venous pressure
d. Decreasing total peripheral resistance
e. Decreasing systemic blood pressure

76. A 42-year-old athlete becomes alarmed when he notices a series of heart palpitations several hours after he exercises. After examining the patient's ECG, the physician notes a sinus rhythm with occasional PVCs (premature ventricular complexes). The physician tells his patient that the palpitations are due to interpolated beats and that they are not a cause for alarm. The benign PVCs occur because of the patient's

a. Prolonged PR interval
b. Bradycardia
c. Depressed ST segment
d. Wide QRS complex
e. Inverted atrial P wave

77. The electrocardiogram is most effective in detecting a decrease in which of the following?

a. Ventricular contractility
b. Mean blood pressure
c. Total peripheral resistance
d. Ejection fraction
e. Coronary blood flow

78. Stroke volume can be increased by which of the following?

a. Decreasing ventricular compliance
b. Increasing venous compliance
c. Decreasing total peripheral resistance
d. Increasing heart rate
e. Decreasing atrial contractility

79. A patient comes to his physician complaining that he is no longer able to exercise as long as he used to. The physician notes crepitant rales (lung sounds), a third heart sound, and normal blood pressure. He sends the patient to cardiology to rule out heart failure. Which one of the following is most consistent with a diagnosis of left heart failure?

a. A decreased heart rate
b. An increased left ventricular wall stress
c. An increased left ventricular ejection fraction
d. A decreased left ventricular energy consumption
e. A decreased pulmonary arterial wedge pressure

80. Which of the following correctly describes an event that normally occurs during the PR interval?

a. The ventricle is contracting
b. The cardiac action potential passes through the AV node
c. There is no change in the voltage tracing on the ECG
d. The mitral and aortic valves are both closed
e. The second heart sound is heard

81. Left ventricular wall stress will be decreased by an increase in which of the following?

a. The left ventricular end-diastolic volume
b. The contractility of the left atrium
c. The thickness of the free wall of the left ventricle
d. The total peripheral resistance
e. The mean arterial blood pressure

82. A 67-year-old female is brought to the emergency room because she fainted at the gym during her daily aerobic workout. A prominent systolic murmur is heard and a presumptive diagnosis of aortic stenosis is made. Which of the following is consistent with that diagnosis?

a. A decreased pulse pressure
b. An increased arterial pressure
c. A decreased left ventricular diastolic pressure
d. An increased ejection fraction
e. A decreased cardiac oxygen consumption

83. The phases of the ventricular muscle action potential are represented by the lettered points on the diagram below. At which point on the ventricular action potential is membrane potential most dependent on calcium permeability?

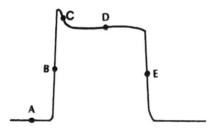

a. Point A
b. Point B
c. Point C
d. Point D
e. Point E

Questions 84–85

Use the following ECG to answer the next two questions.

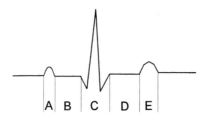

84. During which interval on the above ECG does the aortic valve close?

a. A
b. B
c. C
d. D
e. E

85. During which interval on the ECG does the bundle of His depolarize?

a. A
b. B
c. C
d. D
e. E

86. The diagnosis of a first-degree heart block is made if

a. The PR interval of the ECG is increased
b. The P wave of the ECG is never followed by a QRS complex
c. The P wave of the ECG is sometimes followed by a QRS complex
d. The T wave of the ECG is inverted
e. The ST segment of the ECG is elevated

87. Positive inotropic drugs such a digitalis reduce ischemic cardiac pain (angina) in a dilated failing heart by

a. Decreasing preload
b. Increasing diastolic filling time
c. Decreasing total peripheral resistance
d. Increasing heart rate
e. Increasing coronary blood flow

Questions 88–90

Use the following pressure-volume loop to answer the questions.

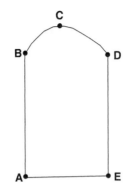

88. The mitral valve opens at point

a. A
b. B
c. C
d. D
e. E

89. The second heart sound begins at point

a. A
b. B
c. C
d. D
e. E

90. Systole begins at point

a. A
b. B
c. C
d. D
e. E

Questions 91–92

Use the following diagram to answer the next two questions.

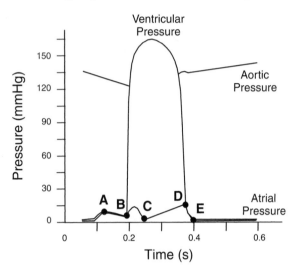

91. Ventricular filling begins at point

a. A
b. B
c. C
d. D
e. E

92. Closing of the mitral valve begins at point

a. A
b. B
c. C
d. D
e. E

93. A 67-year-old man who has difficulty breathing when he exercises makes an appointment to see his physician. Auscultation reveals a systolic murmur leading to the diagnosis of mitral regurgitation. Which of the following laboratory findings is most likely to be present?

a. A decreased arterial pressure
b. An increased pulse pressure
c. A decreased left ventricular preload
d. An increased a wave
e. A decreased cardiac output

94. A 43-year-old male comes to his physician complaining of exhaustion and shortness of breath. After completing the physical exam, the physician suspects the patient may be suffering from cardiac tamponade. Which of the following observations led to the physician's putative diagnosis?

a. Hypertension
b. Bradycardia
c. Third heart sound
d. Pulsus paradoxus
e. Expiratory rales

Questions 95–96

Use the following diagram of three Starling curves to answer the questions.

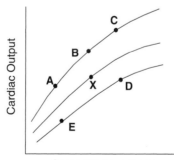

Central Venous Pressure

95. A mild hemorrhage will cause stroke volume to shift from point **X** to point

a. A
b. B
c. C
d. D
e. E

96. An increase in afterload and venous compliance can cause stroke volume to change from the point marked **X** to point

a. A
b. B
c. C
d. D
e. E

97. The upstroke of the SA nodal action potential is produced by opening a channel that is

a. Primarily permeable to Na^+
b. Primarily permeable to Ca^{2+}
c. Primarily permeable to K^+
d. Primarily permeable to Cl^-
e. Equally permeable to Na^+ and K^+

98. The channel responsible for the initiation of phase-4 depolarization in SA nodal cells

a. Is primarily permeable to Na^+
b. Is opened by membrane depolarization
c. Is opened by vagal nerve stimulation
d. Is primarily permeable to K^+
e. Is closed by norepinephrine

99. Sympathetic stimulation of the heart results in which of the following?

a. An increase in the activity of the SR calcium pump
b. An increase in the duration of systole
c. An increase in the duration of diastole
d. A decrease in the affinity of troponin for calcium
e. A decrease in the concentration of Ca^{2+} during systole

100. A 32-year-old female complains of intermittent chest discomfort that occurs most frequently when she drinks lots of coffee to stay up to meet deadlines at work. She is referred to cardiology for an exercise stress test to rule out cardiac ischemia as the cause for her angina. The test will be considered positive if

a. Mean arterial blood pressure increases
b. ST segment depression occurs
c. Tachycardia develops
d. A diastolic murmur is heard
e. The QRS complex widens

Cardiac Physiology

Answers

45. The answer is b. (*Guyton, pp 220–221. Boron, pp 441–444.*) Cardiac output can be measured by using Fick's principle, which asserts that the rate of uptake of a substance by the body (e.g., O_2 consumption in milliliters per minute) is equal to the difference between its concentrations (milliliters per liter of blood) in arterial and venous blood multiplied by the rate of blood flow (cardiac output). This principle is restricted to situations in which arterial blood is the only source of the substance measured. If oxygen consumption by the body at steady state is measured over a period of time and the difference in arterial O_2 and venous O_2 measured by sampling arterial blood and pulmonary arterial blood (which is fully mixed venous blood), cardiac output is obtained from the expression

$$CO = \frac{\dot{V}O_2}{(AO_2 - VO_2)\text{content}}$$

$$CO = \frac{280 \text{ ml/min}}{20 \text{ ml/100 ml} - 12 \text{ ml/100 ml}}$$

$$CO = 3500 \text{ ml/min} = 3.5 \text{ L/min}$$

46. The answer is d. (*Guyton, pp 103–104. Boron, pp 525–528.*) Preload is defined as the sarcomere length at the end of diastole. The parameter most directly related to sarcomere length during this time period is left ventricular end-diastolic volume. Although blood volume, central venous pressure, pulmonary capillary wedge pressure, and left ventricular end-diastolic pressure can all influence preload, they all exert their influence through changes in end-diastolic volume. Each of these parameters could change without altering preload.

47. The answer is b. (*Guyton, pp 104. Boron, 528–530.*) The afterload is the stress on the sarcomeres during the cardiac cycle. According to the law of Laplace (stress = $P \times r$/thickness), the stress is proportional to the pressure (P) and radius (r) and inversely proportional to the thickness of the ventricle during systole. The mean left ventricular systolic pressure would therefore be the best index of afterload. Mean arterial blood pressure (MAP) is normally the same as ventricular pressure and therefore a good index of afterload. However, in a patient with aortic stenosis, the ventricular pressure is higher than the aortic pressure. Although the total peripheral resistance (TPR) can influence afterload by causing changes in mean arterial blood pressure, changes in TPR do not always cause corresponding changes in afterload. For example, during aerobic exercise, afterload (MAP) is often increased, whereas TPR is reduced and following a hemorrhage, TPR is high, whereas afterload (MAP) is low. Pulmonary capillary wedge pressure and left ventricular end-diastolic pressure are estimates of the volume of blood in the ventricle during diastole and are indices of preload.

48. The answer is e. (*Guyton, pp 226–228. Boron, pp 562–564.*) Blood flow through the coronary vessels of the left ventricle is determined by the ratio of perfusion pressure to vascular resistance. The perfusion pressure is directly related to the aortic pressure at the ostia of the coronaries. Myocardial vascular resistance is significantly influenced by the contractile activity of the ventricle. During systole, when the ventricle is contracting, vascular resistance increases substantially. Flow is highest just at the beginning of diastole because, during this phase of the cardiac cycle, aortic pressure is still relatively high and vascular resistance is low due to the fact that the coronary vessels are no longer being squeezed by the contracting myocardium.

49. The answer is d. (*Guyton, pp 134–136. Boron, pp 499–562, 579–582.*) Syncope (fainting) is caused by an inadequate blood flow to the brain. Third-degree heart block occurs when conduction of the action potential from the atria to the ventricles fails all the time. Under these conditions, pacemaker cells within the His-Purkinje system or the ventricular muscle determine the heart rate. Although the heart rate may be high enough to adequately perfuse the brain under resting conditions, a missed beat or a decrease in TPR can lead to a sudden fall in blood pressure leading to syncope. Sinus arrhythmia is a change of the heart rate produced by the normal variation in the rate of phase 4 depolarization of the SA nodal pacemaker cells. First-degree heart block is defined as a higher-than-normal PR interval (greater than 0.2 s). Second-degree heart block occurs when the action potential fails to reach the ventricles some, but not all, of the time. Tachycardia is a heart rate above 100 beats per minute.

50. The answer is c. (*Guyton, pp 134–136. Boron, pp 499–562, 579–582.*) Conduction abnormalities can produce first-degree, second-degree, or third-degree heart block. In a second-degree heart block a P wave is not always followed by a QRS complex as in trace C, where the second P wave is not followed by a QRS complex. In a first-degree heart block, trace D, the interval between the beginning of the P wave and the beginning of the QRS complex (the PR interval) is longer than normal (greater than 0.2 seconds). In a third-degree heart block, conduction between the atria and ventricles is completely blocked so the atrial beats (represented by the P waves) and the ventricular beats (represented by the QRS complex) are completely dissociated.

51. The answer is d. (*Guyton, pp 120–122. Boron, p 498.*) The mean electrical axis (MEA) represents the average direction traveled by the ventricular muscle action potentials as they propagate through the heart. The propagation path and the mass of tissue through which the action potentials travel influence the MEA. The MEA is approximately perpendicular to the axis of the limb lead with the smallest QRS wave magnitude. In this case, the smallest deflection is in lead III. Therefore, the MEA lies along lead aVR. Because the QRS complex is positive in aVR, the MEA is approximately 30 degrees. Because the QRS complex is greater in lead II than in lead I, the MEA is between +60 degrees and +30 degrees.

52. The answer is c. (*Guyton, pp 99–102. Boron, pp 509–513.*) The pressure gradient between regions of the cardiovascular system is directly proportional to the resistance of the intervening structures. During ventricular ejection, the aortic valves are open and do not offer any significant resistance to blood flow. Therefore, there is very little, if any, pressure difference between the left ventricle and the aorta. Because the tricuspid valve is closed during ventricular ejection, there is an appreciable pressure difference between the right ventricle and the left atrium, although this pressure difference is opposite in direction to the flow of blood through the circulatory system. Although pulmonary vascular resistance is relatively small compared with systemic vascular resistance, it nonetheless produces a pressure drop between the right ventricle and the left atrium. Because most of the resistance in the systemic vasculature occurs at the level of the arterioles, there is a large pressure gradient between the aorta and the capillaries.

53. The answer is a. (*Guyton, pp 248–249. Boron, pp 431, 509.*) Blood leaks from the aorta into the left ventricle during diastole in patients with regurgitant aortic valves producing a diastolic murmur. The rapid flow of blood into the left ventricle during diastole also causes an increase in end diastolic volume (preload), which results in a larger stroke volume and therefore, a larger pulse pressure. Typically, mean blood pressure remains the same so the larger pulse pressure is accompanied by an increased systolic and decreased diastolic presure. If too much of the stroke volume flows back into the heart during diastole, mean blood pressure will fall and the baroreceptor reflex will cause an increase in heart rate.

54. The answer is a. (*Guyton, pp 218–220. Boron, pp 227–228, 550–552.*) Stroke volume depends on preload, afterload, and contractility. Decreasing venous compliance forces more blood into the ventricle, resulting in an increased preload and an increased stroke volume. Increasing afterload and decreasing contractility decreases stroke volume. An increase in heart rate may result in a decreased filling time and, therefore, a decrease in preload and stroke volume. A decrease in coronary blood flow causes a decrease in ventricular contractility and stroke volume.

55. The answer is b. (*Guyton, pp 216–219. Boron, pp 550–554.*) Preload is the volume of blood within the ventricles at the end of diastole. A decrease in heart rate increases the time between heartbeats, which allows more blood to enter the left ventricle during diastole. Decreasing blood volume or increasing venous capacitance (compliance) decreases the preload. An increase in TPR or an increase in contractility will decrease preload.

56. The answer is d. (*Guyton, pp 109–111. Boron, pp 488–493.*) The most rapid conduction of the action potential occurs through the Purkinje fibers. The slowest conduction occurs in the AV node. Pacemaker cells located within the SA node initiate the cardiac action potential normally. The action potential propagates from the SA node into the atrial muscle fibers. It then passes through the AV node and the His-Purkinje network to the ventricular muscle fibers. The rapid conduction of the action potential through the His-Purkinje network ensures rapid and synchronous activation of the entire ventricular muscle. The slow conduction through the AV node produces a delay between atrial and ventricular systole, allowing the ventricle to receive the blood ejected by the atria before it contracts.

57. The answer is b. *(Guyton, pp 241–243. Boron, pp 530–533.)* The most obvious deleterious effect of a failing heart is the inability to pump enough blood to satisfy the energy requirements of all the tissues. Among the compensatory mechanisms that develop in response to heart failure is an increase in retention of fluid by the kidney. Increased retention of fluid causes the end-diastolic volume of the heart to increase, which, by the Starling mechanism, increases the strength of the heartbeat. However, two deleterious effects result from an increase in end-diastolic volume. A larger-than-normal end-diastolic volume causes an increase in end-diastolic pressure, which can lead to pulmonary edema. In addition, the large end-diastolic volume increases the wall stress that must be developed by the heart with each beat, and this increases the myocardial requirement of oxygen. The increase in contractility that results from the administration of a positive inotropic drug such as digoxin will allow the heart to produce the same force at a lower volume and thus eliminate the need for an increase in volume of fluid.

58. The answer is b. *(Guyton, pp 100–103. Boron, p 521.)* The ejection fraction (EF) is equal to the stroke volume (SV) divided by the end-diastolic volume (EDV)

$$EF = \frac{SV}{EDV} = \frac{EDV - ESV}{EDV}$$

The stroke volume (SV) is equal to the end diastolic volume (EDV) − end systolic volume (ESV). The end diastolic volume is 150 ml, and the end systolic volume is 60 ml. Therefore the ejection fraction is

$$\frac{130 \text{ mL} - 60 \text{ mL}}{130 \text{ mL}} = 0.55$$

59. The answer is c. *(Guyton, pp 102–103. Boron, pp 522–523.)* Diastolic pressure is the lowest pressure observed in the aorta during each cardiac cycle. It occurs at the end of isovolumic contraction, just before ejection of blood from the left ventricle begins. In this case, isovolumic contraction ends when the pressure within the ventricle rises to 70 mmHg. The term diastolic pressure always refers to arterial blood pressure. In the diagram, the left ventricular end-diastolic pressure equals 5 mmHg.

60. The answer is d. *(Guyton, pp 99–103. Boron, pp 508–513.)* Closure of the semilunar valves (aortic and pulmonic valves) marks the beginning of the isovolumetric relaxation phase of the cardiac cycle. During this brief period (approximately 0.06 s), the ventricles are closed and myocardial relaxation, which began during protodiastole, continues. Intraventricular pressure falls rapidly, although ventricular volume changes little. When intraventricular pressure falls below atrial pressure, the mitral and tricuspid valves open and rapid filling of the ventricles begins.

61. The answer is b. *(Guyton, pp 100–103, 125–127.)* If the QRS complex is positive in lead II, the MEA must be between 30° and +150°. If the QRS complex is positive in a VF, the MEA must be between 0° and 180°. If the QRS complex is negative in lead III, the MEA must be between −150° and +30°. For all three conditions to exist, the MEA must be between 0° and +30°.

62. The answer is b. *(Guyton, pp 141–142. Boron, p 498.)* Atrial fibrillation is an arrhythmia in which the electrical activity of the atrium becomes disorganized and therefore unable to produce a coordinated atrial contraction. The absence of an atrial pulse reduces the emptying of the atria during diastole and results in an enlarged left atrium and increased left atrial pressure. The venous A wave represents atrial contraction and disappears due to the absence of an atrial beat. Decreased filling of the heart results in a decrease in stroke volume. Heart rate increases because the continuous electrical activity of the atria initiates a high rate of ventricular activity. Systemic blood pressure typically falls because of inadequate filling of the ventricles and the resulting decrease in stroke volume.

63. The answer is c. *(Guyton, pp 545–547. Boron, pp 513, 521.)* The second heart sound (S_2) is associated with the closing of the aortic and pulmonic valves. The aortic valve normally closes slightly before the pulmonic valve, resulting in a splitting of the second heart sound into two components. During inspiration the closing of the pulmonic valve is delayed, resulting in a prolongation of the interval between the two components of the second heart sound. During inspiration, the preload on the right heart is increased, resulting in a larger stroke volume. The increased stroke volume causes the delay in the closing of the pulmonic valve. Closure of the mitral valve and tricuspid valves are associated with the first heart sound (S_1).

64. The answer is b. (*Guyton, p 246. Boron, pp 511–513.*) The third heart sound (S_3) is commonly heard in children and young adults and is associated with the filling of the left ventricle. It is also heard in conditions such as heart failure or cardiac tamponade when the compliance of the left ventricle is reduced. It can also occur when rapid filling of the ventricle is abnormally high, for example, in anemia or mitral regurgitation.

65. The answer is c. (*Guyton, pp 213–214. Boron, p 599.*) The magnitude of the cardiac output is regulated to maintain an adequate blood pressure and to deliver an adequate supply of oxygen to the tissues. In anemia, a greater cardiac output is required to supply oxygen to the tissues because the oxygen-carrying capacity of the blood is reduced. In aortic regurgitation, the stroke volume will be increased. However, a portion of the blood ejected by the heart will return to the heart during diastole. Thus, the output delivered to the tissues does not increase despite the fact that the blood ejected by the heart has increased. In hypertension, third-degree heart block, and cardiac tamponade (decreased filling of the heart due to accumulation of fluid within the pericardium), cardiac output will be normal, or, if compensation is not possible, cardiac output will be reduced.

66. The answer is d. (*Guyton, p 103. Boron, pp 523–524.*) Efficiency is defined as work divided by energy consumption. The heart represented by pressure-volume curve 1 in the diagram has a lower end-diastolic volume and, therefore, ejects blood at a lower wall stress than the heart, represented by pressure-volume curve 2. Cardiac energy consumption is directly related to wall stress. Because both hearts eject the same amount of blood (stroke volume) at the same pressure, they perform the same amount of work.

67. The answer is b. (*Guyton, pp 157–159, 247–248. Boron, pp 431, 519.*) A systolic murmur occurs when blood leaks back into the ventricle through an incompetent pulmonic or aortic valve during diastole or travels through a stenotic mitral or tricuspid (AV) valve during ventricular filling. The higher-than-normal height of the jugular blood column reflects an increased right atrial pressure. The combination of a systolic murmur and high right atrial pressure is indicative of regurgitation through the tricuspid valve. Mitral stenosis and aortic regurgitation produce a diastolic murmur.

68. The answer is a. (*Guyton, pp 701, 708.*) Although the cause of her syncope is not given in the history, it is presumably produced by an abnormally slow heart rate due to increased release of ACh by the vagus nerve or by ACh agonists such as muscarine, which is found in certain mushrooms. Atropine blocks the ACh receptors on the SA and AV node, leading to an increased heart rate. The increased heart rate causes blood pressure to increase, relieving her symptoms.

69. The answer is a. (*Guyton, pp 224–226. Boron, pp 1252–1253.*) During exercise, increased oxygen consumption and increased venous return to the heart, resulting in an increase in cardiac output and an increase in blood flow to both skeletal muscle and the coronary circulation, where oxygen utilization is greatest. The increase in cardiac output is due to an increase in both heart rate and stroke volume. Systemic arterial pressure also increases in response to the increase in cardiac output. However, the fall in total peripheral resistance, which is caused by dilation of the blood vessels within the exercising muscles, results in a decrease in diastolic pressure. The pulmonary vessels undergo passive dilation as more blood flows into the pulmonary circulation. As a result, pulmonary vascular resistance decreases. The decrease in venous compliance, caused by sympathetic stimulation, helps maintain ventricular filling during diastole.

70. The answer is a. (*Guyton, pp 107–109. Boron, pp 488–489.*) Phase-4 depolarization is caused by the activation of a Na^+ channel. The channel is called the funny channel because it is activated when the membrane hyperpolarizes in contrast to the Na channel responsible for the action potential, which is activated when the cell depolarizes. Potassium conductance decreases during phase-4 depolarization and thus the flow of potassium out of the cell is diminished. However, this change in potassium current is not responsible for phase-4 depolarization. Chloride conductance does not change during phase 4. The Na/Ca exchanger maintains low intracellular calcium at rest and may reverse its direction and pump calcium into the cell during phase 2 of the cardiac action potential. However, neither the Na/Ca exchanger nor the Na-K pump is involved in phase-4 depolarization.

71. The answer is b. (*Guyton, pp 245–247. Boron, pp 511–513.*) Normal splitting of the second heart sound occurs because the aortic valve (A2) closes before the pulmonic valve (P2). The splitting will be reversed by any condition that delays the closing of the aortic valve. Although the most common cause of reversed splitting is left bundle branch block in which activation of the left ventricle is delayed, reversed splitting can also be caused by any condition in which left ventricular ejection is prolonged. In this case the fatigue and dyspnea are consistent with heart failure caused by a decrease in left ventricular contractility. An increase in right ventricular preload, such as normally occurs during inspiration, will prolong the duration of right ventricular ejection, leading to a prolongation of the normal splitting of the second heart sound.

72. The answer is d. (*Guyton, p 192. Boron, pp 561–562.*) If intracranial pressure is rapidly elevated, cerebral blood flow is reduced. The increase in intracranial pressure stimulates the vasomotor center and produces an increase of systemic blood pressure that may lead to a restoration of cerebral blood flow (Cushing response). A profound bradycardia is also associated with this response. Exercise increases blood pressure and heart rate. Although tissue hypoxia causes arteriolar dilatation, acute hypoxia associated with sudden exposure to high altitudes generates hypertension, as well as excitement, disorientation, and headache. Fever produces tachycardia; blood pressure changes associated with increased body temperature depend on the cause of the temperature. With exercise and increased heat production (and increased blood pressure), vessels dilate in an attempt to dissipate heat. Fever with septic shock will, of course, be associated with a blood pressure decrease owing to vasodilation by endotoxin. Hemorrhage will cause a reflex sympathetic discharge that results in tachycardia and increased total peripheral resistance. If compensation is adequate, blood pressure may not fall.

73. The answer is e. (*Guyton, pp 224–226. Boron, pp 582–585.*) During exercise, sympathetic stimulation of the heart and circulating epinephrine cause an increase in ventricular contractility and heart rate, leading to an increase in cardiac output. Sympathetic stimulation also causes constriction of the venous vessels, which tends to increase end-diastolic volume. Despite sympathetic stimulation of the resistance vessels, local metabolites produced by the exercising muscles cause small arterioles within the muscles to dilate, which produces a decrease in total peripheral resistance (TPR). However, the fall in TPR does not normally produce a drop in mean systemic blood pressure because the increase in cardiac output is sufficient to counteract the fall in resistance. The increased vascular resistance from sympathetic stimulation of the nonexercising muscles and other organs tends to increase TPR and decrease cardiac output.

74. The answer is e. (*Guyton, pp 239–241, 449.*) Orthopnea or dyspnea associated with lying down is caused by redistribution of blood from the periphery to the chest, leading to an increase in pulmonary capillary pressure. Pulmonary capillary pressure is elevated in patients with heart failure. When the patient lies down, the pulmonary capillary pressure is increased, causing the orthopnea. A third heart sound is often heard in heart failure and when associated with a high heart rate produces a gallop rhythm. The third heart sound can also be heard in patients with cor pulmonale (an enlargement of the right heart) and constrictive pericarditis. Neither, however, produces orthopnea. Mitral regurgitation can produce dyspnea but is not associated with a third heart sound.

75. The answer is b. (*Guyton, pp 103–106. Boron, pp 527–533.*) Stroke volume is determined by preload, afterload, and contractility. Increasing heart rate decreases the time for filling during diastole and may decrease preload and therefore stroke volume. Increasing preload by increasing central venous pressure will increase stroke volume. Similarly, decreasing afterload by decreasing total peripheral resistance or systemic blood pressure will cause an increase in stroke volume. Increasing contractility will also increase stroke volume.

76. The answer is b. (*Guyton, pp 137–138. Boron, pp 505–506.*) A premature ventricular beat originates from ventricular pacemaker cells. Most often, these pacemaker cells are reset with each heart beat and therefore do not produce ventricular activation. However, when the sinus rhythm is very slow (bradycardia), there is time for these pacemaker cells to reach threshold and produce a ventricular contraction. Because the patient is a well-trained athlete his bradycardia is an index of his good aerobic conditioning and not a cause for alarm. If the ECG revealed a depressed ST segment, which is a sign of ventricular ischemia, the PVCs could have serious consequences. Although an inverted atrial wave can occur following a PVC (if the action potentials propagate into the atria) and a wide QRS complex, these are results, not causes of the premature contractions.

77. The answer is e. (*Guyton, pp 128–130. Boron, p 501.*) Abnormalities in coronary blood flow resulting in ischemia of the ventricular muscle will lead to a current of injury, which is reflected as an upward or downward shift in the ST segment of the ECG recording. The electrical activity of the heart does not reflect changes in ventricular contractility, blood pressure, ejection fraction, or total peripheral resistance, although all of these can be altered by changes in coronary blood flow.

78. The answer is c. (*Guyton, pp 211–213, 524–530.*) Stroke volume is influenced by ventricular preload, afterload, and contractility. Decreasing total peripheral resistance may result in a decrease in afterload and therefore an increase in stroke volume. Decreasing ventricular compliance (making the heart stiffer) or increasing venous compliance will decrease ventricular filling and, therefore, preload and stroke volume. Similarly, increasing heart rate and deceasing atrial contractility will decrease filling and stroke volume.

79. The answer is b. (*Guyton, pp 235–236. Boron, pp 457–458, 523–524.*) When the left ventricle fails, preload (left ventricular end-diastolic volume) is increased in an attempt to normalize stroke volume. The increase in radius of the dilated ventricle increases wall stress according to the Laplace relationship, $S = \frac{P \times r}{th}$ where S = stress, P = systolic pressure, r = ventricular radius and th = ventricular wall stress. The increase in wall stress requires an increase in energy consumption. The increase in preload increases the left ventricular end-diastolic pressure. Since the pulmonary capillaries are supplying the blood to the left ventricle, an increase in left ventricular end-diastolic pressure must be accompanied by an increase in pulmonary capillary hydrostatic pressure. The decrease in left ventricular contractility associated with heart failure causes the ejection fraction to decrease. Heart rate will be increased by the increased sympathetic nerve activity that accompanies heart failure.

80. The answer is b. (*Guyton, pp 522–524. Boron, pp 498–499.*) The PR interval starts at the beginning of the P wave and ends at the beginning of the QRS complex. The physiologic events that occur during this time period include atrial depolarization, which is responsible for the P wave, AV nodal depolarization, and depolarization of the bundle of His and the Purkinje fibers. SA nodal depolarization precedes the P wave. Since the mass of the SA node is so small, this event cannot be detected on the standard ECG recording. The mitral and aortic valves are closed during isovolemic contraction, which occurs after the QRS complex has begun. The second heart sound occurs at the end of systole.

81. The answer is c. (*Guyton, pp 235–236. Boron, pp 457–458, 523–524.*) The factors that influence wall stress are given by the Laplace relationship ($WS = [P \times r]$/thickness), where P equals the transmural pressure across the wall of the ventricle, r, the radius of the ventricle (determined by end-diastolic volume), and thickness, the thickness of the ventricular wall. Wall stress is reduced if the wall thickness increases. Increasing the systolic pressure developed by the heart (ventricular transmural pressure) or increasing the end-diastolic volume will increase wall stress. Wall stress will also be increased if total peripheral resistance is increased or mean arterial blood pressure is increased because, under both conditions, the heart will have to develop more pressure.

82. The answer is a. (*Guyton, pp 154, 246–247. Boron, pp 431, 508–511.*) In aortic stenosis, the resistance of the aortic valve increases, making it more difficult for blood to be ejected from the heart. Because a pressure drop occurs over the stenotic aortic valve, the ventricular pressure is much larger than the aortic pressure. Although stroke volume typically decreases, leading to a decrease in pulse pressure, a normal cardiac output and arterial pressure can still be maintained by increasing heart rate. However, the increased afterload will lead to a decreased ejection fraction and increased cardiac oxygen consumption.

83. The answer is d. (*Guyton, pp 97–98. Boron, pp 486–488.*) The plateau phase (phase 2) is the result of the influx of calcium. Although calcium channels begin to open during the upstroke (phase 0), the greatest number of calcium channels is open during the plateau. The upstroke is primarily dependent on the opening of Na channels. The initial repolarization (phase 1) is dependent on the inactivation of Na$^+$ channels and the opening of a transient K$^+$ channel. Repolarization (phase 3) is produced by the inactivation of Ca^{2+} channels and the activation of the delayed rectifier K$^+$ channels.

84–85. The answers are 84-e, 85-b. (*Guyton, pp 99–100. Boron, pp 511–513.*) The aortic valve closes when the pressure within the ventricle falls below the pressure within the aorta. This occurs when the ventricular muscle begins to relax. Relaxation begins at the end of the ventricular action potential, which is represented by the T wave (segment **E**) on the ECG recording.

The bundle of His depolarizes during the PR segment (segment **E**), that is, during the interval between the end of atrial depolarization and the beginning of ventricular depolarization. Segment **A**, the P wave, represents atrial depolarization, segment **C**, the QRS complex, represents ventricular depolarization, and segment **D**, the ST segment, represents the time interval during which all of the ventricular muscle is depolarized.

86. The answer is a. (*Guyton, pp 135–136. Boron, pp 502–504.*) The PR interval represents the time it takes for the cardiac action potential to propagate from the SA node to the ventricular muscle. A delay in this interval, normally produced by a slowing in the conduction velocity through the AV node, is called a first-degree heart block. A second-degree heart block occurs when the action potential does not always propagate through the SA node. This produces an uneven heart beat. A third-degree block occurs when the action potential never reaches the ventricle. Under these conditions, pacemakers within the ventricle produce ventricular contraction but the rate is very slow. Inversion of the T wave and elevation of the ECG are indicators of membrane potential defects within the ventricular muscle.

87. The answer is a. (*Guyton, pp 235–238. Boron, pp 457–458, 523–524.*) Ischemic cardiac pain is produced when oxygen demand is greater than the oxygen that can be delivered by the coronary arteries. Positive inotropic agents reduce oxygen demand by increasing cardiac contractility. Although under normal circumstances an increase in contractility will increase oxygen demand, in a dilated heart, it actually decreases oxygen demand. The increase in contractility allows the heart to generate adequate force without increasing preload as much. As a result, the volume of the heart is reduced. Reducing volume decreases wall stress, because, according to the law of Laplace, the wall stress is proportional to the product of force and radius (which is proportional to ventricular volume).

88–90. The answers are 88-a, 89-b, 90-e. (*Guyton, pp 101–103. Boron, pp 522–524, 530–533.*) The left ventricular pressure-volume loop represents the changes in pressure and volume that occur during a cardiac cycle. Point **A** represents the end of the isovolumic relaxation phase and the beginning of the filling phase. At the point the pressure in the left ventricle falls below that in the left atrium, the mitral valve opens and blood begins to flow into the left ventricle. Point **B** represents the end of the ejection phase. At this point, the pressure in the left ventricle falls below the pressure in the aorta, and the aortic valve closes. The retrograde flow of blood against the closed aortic valve produces the second heart sound. Point **E** represents the end of the filling phase and the beginning of the isovolumic contraction phase. At this point, the pressure in the left ventricle increases above the pressure in the left atrium, causing the mitral valve to close. The retrograde flow of blood against the closed mitral valve produces the first heart sound. Systole is defined as the period between the first and second heart sounds and includes the isovolumic contraction and ejection phases. Aortic pressure continues to fall during the isovolumic contraction phase so that the rise in aortic blood pressure (which begins at point **D**) lags behind the beginning of systole.

91–92. The answers are 91-d, 92-a. (*Guyton, pp 99–103. Boron, pp 508–513.*) The graph accompanying the questions illustrates the development of pressure in the aorta, the left atrium, and the left ventricle during a single cardiac cycle. At point **D**, the pressure within the left ventricle is less than the pressure in the left atrium, and, therefore, the mitral valve opens and ventricular filling begins. Although the volume in the left ventricle is increasing, the pressure is falling. During this time period, the recoil of the ventricle causes its pressure to decrease as it is filling. Later in diastole, the pressure of the blood returning from the lungs causes both volume and pressure in the ventricle to increase. At point **A**, the ventricle begins to contract, raising its pressure above that in the atrium and closing the mitral valve. The aortic valve opens at point **B** and closes at point **C**.

93. The answer is d. *(Guyton, pp 99, 156–157, 247–248. Boron, pp 511–512.)* The a wave is the increase in central venous pressure that normally occurs during atrial contraction. Mitral regurgitation will produce a greater atrial preload and therefore a greater force of contraction. The increased atrial volume produces an increased ventricular preload. Blood pressure is typically normal in patients with mitral regurgitation. The greater left ventricular preload produces a greater-than-normal stroke volume. However, the forward stroke volume, the volume entering the aorta, does not increase, so there is no increase in pulse pressure or cardiac output.

94. The answer is d. *(Guyton, pp 214, 231.)* Cardiac tamponade is a disorder of the heart in which an increase in the volume of pericardial fluid compresses the heart and reduces ventricular filling during diastole. Pulsus paradoxus is a clinical sign in which there is an abnormally large decrease (greater than 10 mmHg) in systolic pressure during inspiration. The drop in systolic pressure normally occurs during inspiration because the decreased intrathoracic pressure reduces the flow of blood from the lungs to the left ventricle. The decrease in intrathoracic pressure also increases venous return to the right ventricle. The decrease in ventricular filling during inspiration is exacerbated in cardiac tamponade because the increased volume of blood in the right ventricle cannot push out the right ventricular wall because of the increased fluid in the pericardial space. Instead, the blood pushes against the intraventricular septum, greatly reducing the volume of blood that can enter the left ventricle.

95–96. The answers are 95-a, 96-c. *(Guyton, pp 214–220. Boron, pp 550–554, 585–588.)* Starling's law of the heart states that increasing preload increases the force of contraction. The curves shown in the diagram illustrate that relationship by plotting stroke volume as a function of end-diastolic volume. The Starling curve above the one on which the **X** is marked will result from an increase in contractility or a decrease in afterload. The Starling curve below the one on which the **X** is marked will result from a decrease in contractility or an increase in afterload. A mild hemorrhage, which causes a decrease in blood volume and pressure, will evoke the baroreceptor reflex, which produces an increase in contractility and an increase in heart rate. The increase in heart rate indicates that the new stroke volume will be on the upper curve. The low blood volume and increased heart rate causes a decrease in end-diastolic volume. Therefore, the stroke volume will be at the point marked **A.** An increase in afterload indicates that the new stroke volume will be on the lower curve. The increase in venous compliance results in a decrease in end-diastolic volume, and, therefore, the stroke volume will be at the point marked **C.**

97. The answer is a. (*Guyton, pp 107–109. Boron, pp 486–492.*) Opening the L-type calcium channel produces the upstroke of the SA nodal action potential. This is the same channel that is responsible for the plateau phase of the ventricular action potential. The SA nodal cells have very few of the Na^+ channels that open during the upstroke of the ventricular action potential. And because the maximum diastolic potential of the SA nodal cells is approximately −60 mV, any sodium channels that may be expressed on their cell membrane will be inactivated.

98. The answer is a. (*Guyton, pp 107–109. Boron, pp 486–492.*) The funny channel produces phase-4 depolarization of the SA nodal cells, which is permeable to Na^+. The channel is called a funny channel because, unlike most Na^+ channels, which open when the cell is depolarized, this channel is activated when the cell is polarized. It therefore opens at the end of the previous action potential, allowing Na^+ to flow through the cell membrane and depolarize the cell. Vagal stimulation slows the heart rate by hyperpolarizing the SA node (by opening K^+ channels) and by slowing the rate of phase-4 depolarization (by making it more difficult for the funny channels to open). Norepinephrine increases the heart rate by increasing the rate at which the funny channels open, increasing the rate of phase-4 depolarization.

99. The answer is a. (*Guyton, pp 111–113. Boron, pp 492–493.*) Sympathetic stimulation of the heart activates a G protein, which, by activating adenylyl cyclase, increases the intracellular concentration of cAMP. cAMP activates protein kinase A, which phosphorylates a number of proteins, including phospholamban. Unphosphorylated phospholamban inhibits the SR Ca^{2+} pump. Inhibition of the SR Ca^{2+} pump is removed when phospholamban is phosphorylated, and, therefore, its activity is increased. The increased activity of the SR Ca^{2+} pump removes Ca^{2+} from the cytoplasm rapidly and therefore reduces the duration of systole. Sympathetic stimulation of the heart also increases heart rate. Therefore, the total duration of the cardiac cycle is decreased, resulting in a decrease in systole and diastole. Because the duration of systole is reduced disproportionately by the phosphorylation of phospholamban, the decrease in diastole is not as great as might be, predicted by the increase in heart rate, and, therefore, diastolic filling is not compromised. Sympathetic stimulation increases the amount of Ca^{2+} released from the SR during systole and decreases the affinity of troponin for Ca^{2+}. The increase in systolic Ca^{2+} concentration overcomes the deceased affinity of troponin for Ca^{2+}, resulting in an increased contractility.

100. The answer is b. (*Guyton, pp 128–130. Boron, pp 498–502.*) A stress test is conducted by asking a patient to increase his or her exercise intensity while monitoring blood pressure and the electrical activity of the heart. Ischemia occurs if the myocardial oxygen demand brought about by the increased exercise intensity is not matched by an increase in myocardial blood flow. An ischemic episode is indicated by an ST segment depression. Mean arterial blood pressure and heart rate normally rise. The presence of a diastolic murmur or conduction abnormalities in the ECG are not diagnostic of ischemic heart disease. The exercise test will also be terminated if dizziness, dyspnea, or ventricular tachycardia develop or if blood pressure falls.

Vascular Physiology

Questions

DIRECTIONS: Each question below contains five suggested responses. Select the **one best** response to each question.

101. After a mild hemorrhage, compensatory responses initiated by the baroreceptor reflex keeps blood pressure at or close to its normal value. Which of the following values is less after compensation for the hemorrhage than it was before the hemorrhage?

a. Venous compliance
b. Heart rate
c. Ventricular contractility
d. Total peripheral resistance
e. Coronary blood flow

102. The constriction of a blood vessel to one-half of its resting diameter would increase its resistance to blood flow by a factor of

a. 2
b. 4
c. 8
d. 12
e. 16

103. During aerobic exercise, blood flow remains relatively constant within

a. The skin
b. The heart
c. The brain
d. The skeletal muscles
e. The kidneys

104. Which of the following conditions causes pulse pressure to increase?

a. Tachycardia
b. Hypertension
c. Hemorrhage
d. Aortic stenosis
e. Heart failure

105. Sudden standing evokes the baroreceptor reflex. Which of the following will be greater after a person suddenly stands up than it was before the person stood?

a. The end-diastolic volume
b. The renal blood flow
c. The venous return
d. The pulse pressure
e. The ejection fraction

106. A 52-year-old man is brought to the emergency room with severe chest pain. Angiography demonstrates a severe coronary occlusion. A thrombolytic agent is administered to re-establish perfusion. Which of the following does the thrombolytic agent activate?

a. Heparin
b. Plasminogen
c. Thrombin
d. Kininogen
e. Prothrombin

107. Central venous pressure is increased by

a. Decreasing blood volume
b. Increasing venous compliance
c. Increasing total peripheral resistance
d. Decreasing heart rate
e. Decreasing plasma aldosterone concentration

108. Capillary permeability is lowest within the

a. Kidneys
b. Spleen
c. Liver
d. Brain
e. Skin

109. Blood flow through an organ would be increased by decreasing

a. The diameter of the arterial vessels
b. The number of open arterial vessels
c. The arterial pressure
d. The diameter of the venous vessels
e. The hematocrit

110. A 22-year-old woman is hospitalized with a history of severe respiratory distress, fever, and fatigue. ST segment and T wave abnormalities suggest acute viral myocarditis. Over the next several days significant edema develops. The edema is most likely caused by which of the following?

a. Increased heart rate
b. Decreased arterial pressure
c. Increased plasma protein concentration
d. Decreased capillary permeability
e. Increased right atrial pressure

111. A reduction in carotid sinus pressure would cause a decrease in which of the following?

a. Heart rate
b. Myocardial contractility
c. Total peripheral resistance
d. Venous compliance
e. Cardiac output

112. Which of the following organs has the highest arteriovenous O_2 difference under normal resting conditions?

a. Brain
b. Heart
c. Skeletal muscle
d. Kidney
e. Stomach

113. The percentage of the total cardiac output distributed to any single organ is most dependent on

a. The contractile state of the heart
b. The magnitude of mean blood pressure
c. The magnitude of diastolic pressure
d. The ratio of an organ's vascular resistance to total peripheral resistance (TPR)
e. the magnitude of cardiac output

114. At which of the following sites does the blood flow lose the greatest amount of energy?

a. Mitral valve
b. Large arteries
c. Arterioles
d. Capillaries
e. Venules

115. Which of the following decreases during aerobic exercise?
a. Circulating blood volume
b. Heart rate
c. Skin temperature
d. Cerebral blood flow
e. Mean blood pressure

116. A 10-year-old boy is brought to the emergency room after fainting during soccer practice. He often complained that he was tired and had difficulty catching his breath. The presence of a systolic murmur and the ventricular and aortic pressure waves illustrated below suggest which diagnosis?

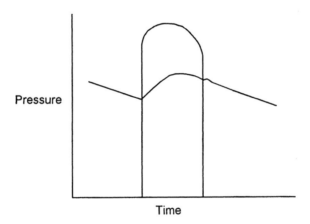

a. Aortic regurgitation
b. Aortic stenosis
c. Congestive heart failure
d. Mitral regurgitation
e. Atherosclerosis

117. Based on the following values, the flow of fluid out of the capillaries will be zero if the average interstitial hydrostatic pressure is

Average capillary hydrostatic pressure = 18 mmHg
Average capillary oncotic pressure = 27 mmHg
Average interstitial oncotic pressure = 7 mmHg

a. −4 mmHg
b. −2 mmHg
c. 0 mmHg
d. +1 mmHg
e. +2 mmHg

118. The graph below illustrates the pressure-volume curves for the arterial and venous systems. The ratio of the arterial compliance to the venous compliance is approximately

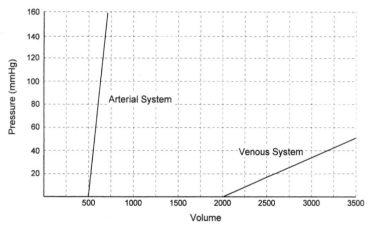

a. 15:1
b. 10:1
c. 1:1
d. 1:10
e. 1:20

119. Which one of the following characteristics is most similar in the systemic and pulmonary circulations?

a. Stroke work
b. Preload
c. Afterload
d. Peak systolic pressure
e. Blood volume

120. Tachycardia and a wide pulse pressure are observed in a 6-year-old girl during a routine physical examination. Echocardiography reveals a patent ductus arteriosus. Which one of the following best describes the function of the ductus arteriosus in the fetal circulation?

a. It prevents the flow of blood into the lungs of the fetus
b. It delivers oxygenated blood from the placenta to the left ventricle
c. It allows blood to flow from the aorta to the pulmonary artery in the fetus
d. It maintains normal fetal blood pressure
e. It is located in the septum between the left and right atrium

121. The following diagram illustrates the relative resistance of three vessels. The ratio of the flow in vessel X to the flow in vessel Y is

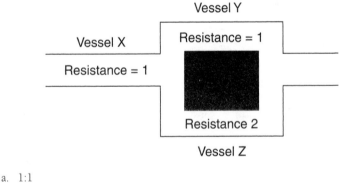

a. 1:1
b. 3:2
c. 2:1
d. 3:1
e. 4:3

122. The data below were obtained from a patient before and after administration of a drug that increased his mean right atrial pressure.

	Before	After
Mean right atrial pressure	8 mmHg	20 mmHg
Mean aortic pressure	80 mmHg	80 mmHg
Cardiac output	4 L/min	5 L/min

The ratio of the patient's total peripheral resistance before administration of the drug to the total peripheral resistance after administration of the drug is

a. 1:1
b. 3:2
c. 4:3
d. 5:4
e. 6:5

123. A 57-year-old man developed severe hypertension after induction of surgical anesthesia and was treated with vasodilators to prevent a potentially life-threatening subendocardial myocardial infarction. At which point in the following diagram of an aortic pressure wave is the patient most at risk for endocardial infarction?

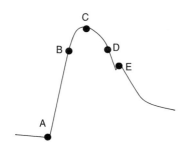

a. A
b. B
c. C
d. D
e. E

124. Which of the following values is greater in the pulmonary circulation than in the systemic circulation?

a. The mean arterial pressure
b. The arterial resistance
c. The vascular compliance
d. The blood flow
e. The sympathetic tone

125. The greatest percentage of blood volume is found in the

a. Heart
b. Aorta
c. Distributing arteries and arterioles
d. Capillaries
e. Venules and veins

126. A 67-year-old woman with a history of venous thromboembolism is placed on warfarin (Coumadin) prophylactically. Bleeding can occur if the blood concentration of Coumadin becomes too high. Should bleeding occur, it can be prevented by the administration of

a. Aspirin
b. Heparin
c. tPA (tissue plasminogen activator)
d. Vitamin K
e. Fibrinogen

127. A 42-year-old patient with a rare blood type is scheduled for surgery that will likely require a transfusion. Because the patient has a rare blood type, an autologous blood transfusion is planned. Prior to surgery, 1500 ml of blood is collected. The collection tubes contain calcium citrate, which prevents coagulation by

a. Blocking thrombin
b. Binding factor XII
c. Binding vitamin K
d. Chelating calcium
e. Activating plasminogen

128. Prior to having his first colonoscopy, a 50-year-old male undergoes a bleeding time test to rule out any clotting disorders. Bleeding time is determined by nicking the skin superficially with a scalpel blade and measuring the time required for hemostasis. It will be markedly abnormal (prolonged) in a person who has

a. Anemia
b. Vitamin K deficiency
c. Leukopenia
d. Thrombocytopenia
e. Hemophilia

129. Soon after delivery a new born baby becomes cyanotic. The cyanosis is not relieved by breathing 100% oxygen. A diagnosis of persistent fetal circulation is made. The clinical signs of persistent fetal circulation are caused by which of the following?

a. Mitral regurgitation
b. Left ventricular hypertrophy
c. Pulmonary vasoconstriction
d. Systemic hypertension
e. Aortic coarctation

130. A 63-year-old woman presented with the acute onset of right eye pain. Ophthalmic and neurologic examinations were normal except for a loud right carotid bruit. The eye pain ceased following carotid endarterectomy. The bruit was most likely caused by

a. A high velocity of blood within the carotid artery
b. An increase in blood viscosity
c. A widening of the carotid artery
d. An increase in hematocrit
e. A lengthening of the carotid artery

131. Systemic arteriolar constriction may result from an increase in the local concentration of which of the following?

a. Nitric oxide
b. Angiotensin II
c. Atrial natriuretic peptide
d. Beta (β) agonists
e. Hydrogen ion

132. A 67-year-old patient underwent endoscopic third ventriculostomy (ETV) to treat his obstructive hydrocephalus. Intracranial pressure increased during the procedure. Which of the following changes in the cardiovascular system was caused by the increased intracranial pressure?

a. A decrease in ventricular contractility
b. A decrease in heart rate
c. A decrease in mean blood pressure
d. A decrease in stroke volume
e. A decrease in total peripheral resistance

133. After an episode of exercise training, the trained individual will have which of the following?

a. A decreased density of mitochondria in the trained muscles
b. An increased resting heart rate
c. A decreased maximum oxygen consumption
d. An increased stroke volume
e. A decreased extraction of oxygen by exercising muscles

134. Which of the following increases during aerobic exercise?

a. Diastolic blood pressure
b. Cerebral vascular resistance
c. Mixed venous oxygen tension
d. Blood flow to the kidney
e. Circulating blood volume

135. Pulse pressure increases when

a. Heart rate increases
b. Stroke volume decreases
c. Aortic compliance increases
d. Aortic stenosis develops
e. Mean arterial pressure increases

136. The distribution of blood among the various organs of the body is regulated by regulating the resistance of the

a. Arteries
b. Arterioles
c. Precapillary sphincters
d. Postcapillary venules
e. Veins

137. Flow of fluid through the lymphatic vessels will be decreased if there is an increase in which of the following?

a. Capillary pressure
b. Capillary permeability
c. Interstitial protein concentration
d. Capillary oncotic pressure
e. Central venous pressure

138. When the EMT arrives at the scene of an automobile accident, she finds a hemorrhaging, unconscious young woman. Which of the following signs would be observed in the victim of the automobile accident?

a. Metabolic alkalosis
b. Dry skin
c. Polyuria
d. Bradycardia
e. Low hematocrit

139. A 37-year-old patient is brought to the emergency room in shock. Treatment is directed toward anaphylactic shock rather than hypovolumic shock because

a. Cardiac output is higher than normal
b. Ventricular contractility is greater than normal
c. Total peripheral resistance is greater than normal
d. Serum creatinine is elevated
e. Heart rate is greater than normal

140. An 82-year-old male reports episodes of lightheadedness whenever he turns his head while backing up his car. A diagnosis of carotid sinus sensitivity is made. His symptoms are caused by an increase in which of the following?

a. Total peripheral resistance
b. Right atrial pressure
c. Venous tone
d. Ventricular contractility
e. Vagal nerve activity

141. A 29-year-old male presents with recurring episodes of edema accompanied by chills and fever. A history reveals prolonged travel in the Far East and a diagnosis of parasites that block the lymph vessels. Which of the following characteristics of vessels is most different when comparing the vascular and lymphatic systems?

a. Spontaneous vasomotor activity
b. Absorption of proteins from the interstitial fluid
c. Absorption of nutrients from the GI tract
d. Backflow of fluid is presented by valves
e. Endothelial cells form the vessel walls

142. During a routine physical examination, a 35-year-old male is found to have a blood pressure of 170/105 mmHg. History reveals episodes of headache accompanied by palpitations, diaphoresis, and anxiety. A tentative diagnosis of pheochromocytoma is confirmed when blood pressure falls in response to the administration of which of the following?

a. A beta agonist
b. An alpha blocker
c. An ACE inhibitor
d. A loop diuretic
e. An AII antagonist

143. A 65-year-old slightly cyanotic male presents to his physician complaining of dizziness and fatigue. A blood test reveals a hematocrit of 62, leading to the diagnosis of polycythemia vera. Treatment consists of periodic phlebotomy to reduce the hematocrit. The reduction in hematocrit is beneficial because it

a. Reduces blood viscosity
b. Increases arterial oxygen saturation
c. Reduces blood pressure
d. Increases cardiac output
e. Decreases oxygen-carrying capacity

Questions 144–146

Use the diagram below to answer the next three questions. The point marked "Control" represents the state of the cardiovascular system in the resting state.

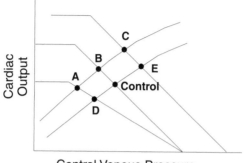

Central Venous Pressure

144. An increase in total peripheral resistance and contractility is represented by a shift from the resting state to point

a. A
b. B
c. C
d. D
e. E

145. Which of the following would be consistent with a shift from the resting state (control) to point B?

a. The person stood up suddenly
b. The person began exercising
c. The person was given a transfusion
d. The person's afterload was increased
e. The person was given a positive inotropic drug

146. Which of the following would be consistent with a shift from the resting state (control) to point E?

a. The person stood up suddenly
b. The person began exercising
c. The person was given a transfusion
d. The person's afterload was increased
e. The person was given a positive inotropic drug

Vascular Physiology

Answers

101. The answer is a. (*Boron, pp 585–590. Guyton, pp 189–190, 254–255.*) The fall in blood volume and pressure produced by hemorrhage elicits the baroreceptor reflex. The reflex increases the activity of the sympathetic nervous system and decreases the activity of the parasympathetic nerves innervating the heart. Sympathetic stimulation of the smooth muscle surrounding the venous vessels decreases their compliance, causing end-diastolic volume (EDV) to increase. However, the EDV does not increase above the levels observed prior to the hemorrhage. Heart rate, ventricular contractility, and total peripheral resistance are all increased above their prehemorrhage levels by sympathetic stimulation. The coronary blood flow increases to meet the increased energy requirements of the heart beating at a higher rate with increased contractility.

102. The answer is e. (*Boron, pp 428–430.*) According to Poiseuille's law, resistance is inversely proportional to the fourth power of the radius $[R \propto (1/r^4)]$. Therefore, if the radius of a blood vessel is decreased by a factor of 2, the resistance to blood flow would increase by a factor of 2^4, or by 16 times.

103. The answer is c. (*Boron, pp 559–562.*) Aerobic exercise causes an increase in sympathetic discharge and circulating catecholamines, which results in an increased heart rate, ventricular contractility, and cardiac output. Blood pressure rises despite the fall in TPR that results from the dilation of the blood vessels providing blood to the exercising skeletal muscle. Blood flow to the gut, the kidneys, and the nonexercising muscles is reduced by sympathetic constriction of the arterioles leading to these organs. Blood flow to the skin is increased to prevent overheating. Coronary blood flow increases to meet the increased metabolic needs of the heart. Blood flow to the brain is kept relatively constant by autoregulatory mechanisms.

104. The answer is b. (*Boron, pp 435–437, 453–462.*) Pulse pressure is proportional to the amount of blood entering the aorta during systole and inversely proportional to aortic compliance. Pulse pressure increases with hypertension because hypertension causes aortic compliance to decrease. Whether the hypertension is a result of an increased cardiac output or an increased peripheral resistance, the higher arterial pressure is caused by an increase in arterial blood volume. The increased blood volume stretches the arterial wall, making it stiffer and decreasing its compliance. Stroke volume is decreased with tachycardia, hemorrhage, and heart failure, reducing pulse pressure in all three cases. In aortic stenosis, the ejection of blood from the ventricle is slowed and the increase in arterial blood volume during systole is less than normal.

105. The answer is e. *(Boron, pp 535–545.)* When a person rises suddenly, blood pools in the dependent portions of the body, causing decreases in venous return, left ventricular end-diastolic volume, stroke volume, and pulse pressure. The reduced stroke volume leads to a drop in cardiac output and, therefore, a drop in blood pressure. Decreased blood pressure produces the baroreceptor reflex, leading to an increase in sympathetic activity, which increases total peripheral resistance, cardiac contractility, heart rate, and ejection fraction. These changes in the cardiovascular system return blood pressure toward normal.

106. The answer is b. *(Boron, pp 425–426. Guyton, pp 420–421.)* Plasminogen is the inactive precursor of plasmin, the proteolytic enzyme involved in clot dissolution. An infusion of tissue plasminogen activator (tPA) soon after a heart attack (and possibly a thrombolytic stroke) can lessen the chances of permanent damage. Thrombin, the enzyme ultimately responsible for the formation of fibrin monomers, is generated from prothrombin by activated factor X. Activation of factor X occurs via both extrinsic and intrinsic pathways. Kininogens are enzymes responsible for the production of peptides (kinins) associated with inflammation. Heparin is an anticlotting agent found on endothelial cell surfaces.

107. The answer is d. *(Boron, pp 550–554. Guyton, pp 215–220.)* Central venous pressure is the hydrostatic pressure in the great veins at their entrance to the right atrium. Increasing venous compliance would decrease pressure in the venous vessels and therefore would decrease central venous pressure. Decreasing blood volume would have the same effect. Reducing the plasma concentration of aldosterone would result in a decrease in blood volume. Increasing total peripheral resistance would tend to shift volume from the venous side of the circulation to the arterial side, resulting in a decrease in venous pressure. Increasing cardiac output tends to lower central venous pressure, whereas lowering cardiac output tends to increase central venous pressure. A reduction in heart rate would tend to lower cardiac output and therefore increase central venous pressure.

108. The answer is d. *(Boron, pp 410, 467–469. Guyton, p 714.)* Capillaries within the brain are continuous capillaries; they do not contain any aqueous pores for diffusion of water-soluble materials. Unlike other continuous capillaries, such as those found in skin and muscle, the gaps between endothelial cells in brain capillaries are closed. These closed gaps make them essentially impermeable to all but fat-soluble materials. The brain's capillaries are the least permeable of all the body's capillaries. The endothelial cells within the kidney are fenestrated. They contain fenestrations, or windows, through which all substances dissolved in the plasma except proteins can diffuse. Capillaries within the spleen and liver are discontinuous. Wide gaps between adjacent capillary endothelial cells allow proteins and cellular elements to easily pass through.

109. The answer is e. *(Boron, pp 426–435. Guyton, pp 150–151.)* Blood flow through an organ is increased by either increasing the perfusion pressure across the organ or by decreasing the vascular resistance. A decrease in the arterial pressure would decrease the perfusion pressure. Decreasing the diameter of the arterial or venous vessels or decreasing the number of open arterial vessels would contribute to increasing vascular resistance. If the hematocrit is decreased, the viscosity of the blood is decreased, resulting in a decrease in resistance and, therefore, an increase in blood flow through an organ.

110. The answer is e. *(Boron, pp 469–475. Guyton, pp 166–170.)* Net filtration from systemic capillaries is dependent on the Starling forces and capillary permeability. The equation is

$$\text{Net Filtration} \propto K_f \times [(P_{\text{capillary}} - P_{\text{tissue}}) - (\pi_{\text{capillary}} - \pi_{\text{tissue}})]$$

Increasing right atrial pressure will increase the filtration of fluid from systemic capillaries, leading to edema. All of the other choices will cause a decrease in filtration.

111. The answer is d. (*Boron, pp 536–545.*) A reduction in carotid sinus pressure due to a decrease in mean blood pressure would elicit a baroreceptor reflex tending to restore blood pressure to normal. The reflex response includes an increase in sympathetic nervous system activity, which would cause an increase in heart rate and myocardial contractility, both of which would tend to increase cardiac output. Sympathetic stimulation would also cause constriction of both the arterioles and venous vessels. Arteriolar constriction would cause an increase in total peripheral resistance. Sympathetic stimulation of the venous vessels would cause a decrease in venous compliance.

112. The answer is b. (*Boron, pp 466–467, 562–564, 673.*) The overall arteriovenous O_2 difference is determined by the oxygen consumption of a tissue and its blood flow. Because of the high rate of metabolism in the heart compared with its blood flow, it has the highest arteriovenous O_2 difference of any major organ of the body under normal conditions. The heart can extract a large amount of oxygen because of its high capillary density. Blood flow to the kidney and skin is far in excess of their metabolic needs, so little oxygen is removed from the blood as it passes through these organs; therefore, their arteriovenous O_2 differences are rather small. Under normal conditions, the arteriovenous O_2 difference in skeletal muscle is quite low. However, this value can increase substantially during vigorous exercise.

113. The answer is d. (*Boron, pp 449–450.*) Arterial vessels arranged in parallel supply the major organs of the body. The relative resistance of each parallel pathway determines the distribution of blood flow through a parallel network of vessels. The ratio of that resistance to the total resistance will determine the percentage of flow going through each of the parallel networks. The other factors mentioned would influence the magnitude of the cardiac output, which is the total amount of blood flowing through the entire system. However, none of these factors have any direct effect on the way blood flow is distributed to the organs of the body.

114. The answer is c. (*Boron, pp 426–428, 451–453.*) The energy imparted to the blood by ventricular systole is dissipated as the blood flows through the circulation. The greatest energy loss occurs where the resistance to blood flow is greatest. This would also be the site of the greatest pressure change. The arteriolar vessels produce the largest resistance to blood, and thus the greatest energy loss and pressure drop occur as the blood passes through them. Normal mitral valves offer almost no resistance to flow and thus there is almost no difference between ventricular pressure and atrial pressure during diastole. This explains why left atrial pressure, as evaluated by pulmonary capillary wedge pressure, can be used as an index of left ventricular end-diastolic pressure in patients with normal mitral valves. Under normal conditions, venous vessels contribute very little to vascular resistance.

115. The answer is a. (*Boron, pp 1252–1254.*) Under normal circumstances, circulating blood volume decreases during aerobic exercise. The decrease in volume is the result of increased filtration of water out of the capillaries within the exercising muscles. Increased filtration occurs because more capillaries within the exercising muscles are filled with blood and the pressure within each capillary is higher. The increased sympathetic activity accompanying the exercise causes an increase in heart rate, which in turn increases the cardiac output. The increase in cardiac output causes an increase in blood pressure, despite the decreased peripheral resistance. The skin temperature increases as more blood is diverted to the skin for the purpose of eliminating the heat generated by the exercising muscles. Brain blood flow is kept constant by autoregulation.

116. The answer is b. (*Boron, pp 431, 509. Guyton, pp 248–249.*) Systolic murmurs are caused by mitral or tricuspid regurgitation or by aortic or pulmonic stenosis. Aortic stenosis increases the resistance of the aortic valve, producing a large pressure drop between the ventricle and aorta. Under normal conditions, the aortic valve offers almost no resistance to flow, and, therefore, there would be virtually no pressure gradient between the left ventricle and the aorta.

117. The answer is b. (*Boron, pp 470–475. Guyton, pp 187, 191–193.*) The movement of fluid through capillaries is governed by hydrostatic pressures and by the capillaries' permeability to water. The hydrostatic pressures are referred to as Starling forces and include the oncotic pressures of the capillary and interstitial proteins and the hydrostatic pressures within the capillary and interstitium. Flow is zero when the sum of the Starling forces equals zero.

$$[(P_{\text{capillary}} - P_{\text{tissue}}) - (\pi_{\text{capillary}} - \pi_{\text{tissue}})] = 0$$

$$[(18 \text{ mmHg} - P_{\text{tissue}}) - (27 \text{ mmHg} - 7 \text{ mmHg})] = 0$$

$$P_{\text{tissue}} = 18 \text{ mmHg} - 27 \text{ mmHg} + 7 \text{ mmHg} = -2 \text{ mmHg}$$

118. The answer is e. *(Boron, pp 453–457. Guyton, pp 152–153.)* Compliance is defined as the change in volume divided by the change in pressure ($\Delta V/\Delta P$). The lower the compliance, the stiffer the vessel becomes. The venous system is much more compliant than the arterial system. The arterial compliance is

$$\text{Arterial compliance} = \frac{\Delta V}{\Delta P} = \frac{250 \text{ mL}}{160 \text{ mmHg}} = 1.56 \text{ mL/mmHg}$$

$$\text{Venous compliance} = \frac{\Delta V}{\Delta P} = \frac{1500 \text{ mL}}{50 \text{ mmHg}} = 30 \text{ mL/mmHg}$$

$$\frac{\text{Arterial compliance}}{\text{Venous compliance}} = \frac{1.56 \text{ mL/mmHg}}{30 \text{ mL/mmHg}} = 1:19.2$$

119. The answer is b. *(Boron, pp 696–699. Guyton, pp 444–446.)* The right and left ventricles are in series with one another so that the entire cardiac output (except for a small anatomic shunt) passes through both circulations. Since the two ventricles beat at the same rate, their stroke volumes are the same. However, the resistance of the pulmonary vasculature is much smaller than that of the systemic circulation; thus, the afterload and stroke work are greater on the left side than on the right side. Because the same cardiac output is ejected into a higher resistance, peak systolic pressure is higher on the left side than on the right side. Only about 10% of the blood volume is within the pulmonary circulation at any one time. About two-thirds of the blood volume is stored within the systemic veins and venules. Although the left and right preloads are not identical, they are very similar.

120. The answer is a. *(Boron, pp 1197–1204. Guyton, pp 249–251, 960–962.)* The ductus arteriosus is a low-resistance arterial vessel of the fetus through which blood flows from the pulmonary artery to the aorta, bypassing the lungs. In fetal life, there is no need for blood to flow through the lungs because blood is oxygenated in the placenta. Soon after birth, the pulmonary vascular resistance falls, allowing blood to flow from the pulmonary artery to the lungs. The high oxygen tension in the blood of the baby causes the resistance of the ductus arteriosus to increase. When the ductus arteriosus does not close at birth, it is called a patent ductus arteriosus. The opening between the left and right atria in the fetus is called the foramen ovale. It, too, normally closes at birth.

121. The answer is b. (*Boron, pp 426–429.*) The ratio of the blood flow through vessels Y and Z is inversely proportional to their resistance. Because vessel Y has half the resistance of vessel Z, it has twice the blood flow. The blood flowing through vessel X is the sum of the blood flowing through vessels Y and Z ($2 + 1 = 3$). Therefore, the ratio of the blood flowing through vessels X and Y is 3:2.

$$Q_{\text{Vessel Y}} \propto \frac{1}{1} \; ; Q_{\text{Vessel Z}} \propto \frac{1}{2}$$

$$\frac{Q_{\text{Vessel Y}}}{Q_{\text{Vessel Z}}} = \frac{1}{1} = \frac{2}{1} \; ;$$

$$Q_{\text{Vessel X}} \propto Q_{\text{Vessel Y}} + Q_{\text{Vessel Z}} \propto 2 + 1 = 3$$

$$\frac{Q_{\text{Vessel X}}}{Q_{\text{Vessel Y}}} \propto \frac{3}{2}$$

122. The answer is b. (*Boron, pp 426–427. Guyton, pp 146–151.*) The relationship between cardiac output (CO), total peripheral resistance (TPR), and blood pressure is

$$\text{Aortic pressure} - \text{right atrial pressure} = \text{CO} \times \text{TPR}$$

$$\text{TPR}_{\text{Before Drug}} = \frac{80 \text{ mmHg} - 8 \text{ mmHg}}{4 \text{ L/min}} = 18 \text{ mmHg/L/min}$$

$$\text{TPR}_{\text{After Drug}} = \frac{80 \text{ mmHg} - 20 \text{ mmHg}}{5 \text{ L/min}} = 12 \text{ mmHg/L/min}$$

$$\frac{\text{TPR}_{\text{Before Drug}}}{\text{TPR}_{\text{After Drug}}} = \frac{18}{12} = 3:2$$

Because the aortic pressure is so much higher-than-normal right atrial pressure, the right atrial pressure is typically ignored when writing the equation so that MBP is set equal to CO × TPR. This simplification is not appropriate when calculating the mean blood pressure in the pulmonary circulation because there is a much smaller difference between the mean pulmonary artery pressure and the left atrial pressure.

123. The answer is a. *(Boron, pp 563–564.)* Subendocardial infarctions are most likely to occur when coronary blood flow is lowest. Coronary blood flow depends on the pressure perfusing the coronary vessels and the compressive forces produced by the contracting ventricles. The coronary blood flow is lowest during isovolumic contraction (point **A,** just before the rise in aortic pressure indicates the end of the isovolumic pressure phase) when the aortic pressure is low and the compressive forces are high. Coronary blood flow increases during ejection, as the perfusing pressure increases. However, the flow is still limited by the compressive forces produced by the contracting ventricle. The greatest coronary blood flow occurs early in diastole, when the ventricle has relaxed and the aortic perusing pressure is still relatively high.

124. The answer is c. *(Boron, pp 696–699. Guyton, pp 444–446.)* The same amount of blood flows through the pulmonary and systemic circulations. However, the mean blood pressure in the pulmonary circulation is much lower (15 mmHg) compared to the mean blood pressure in the systemic circulation (90 mmHg). The pulmonary blood pressure is lower because the resistance to blood flow in the pulmonary circulation is much lower than the resistance to blood flow in the systemic circulation. In addition, the pulmonary blood vessels are more compliant than the systemic blood vessels. Therefore, although the stroke volume of the left and right ventricles is the same, the pulse pressure in the pulmonary artery (25/10) is lower than that in the aorta (120/80). The resistance of the systemic circulation is determined by the activity of the sympathetic nerves innervating the arteriolar smooth muscle. The smooth muscle surrounding the pulmonary vessels receives very little sympathetic innervation.

125. The answer is e. *(Boron, pp 450–451. Guyton, p 160.)* The total circulating blood volume is approximately 70 mL/kg, about two-thirds of which is found in the systemic veins and venules. A significant volume of blood (15%) is found in the pulmonary circulation. The large volume of blood found on the venous side of the circulation is used to adjust circulating blood volume. For example during hemorrhage, contraction of the veins and venules of the skin increases the amount of blood available for perfusion of the heart and brain.

126. The answer is d. *(Boron, p 1226. Guyton, pp 428–429.)* Warfarin is often prescribed for patients at risk for thromboembolic episodes. Vitamin K is necessary for the conversion of prothrombin to thrombin. Thrombin is an important intermediate in the coagulation cascade. It converts fibrinogen to fibrin and is a powerful activator of platelets. Warfarin interferes with the activity of vitamin K and therefore reduces the likelihood of clot formation. Administering vitamin K can restore coagulation if warfarin therapy leads to excessive bleeding. Heparin prevents clotting by inhibiting thrombin. Aspirin blocks the formation of thromboxane A_2, which is necessary for platelet aggregation. Tissue plasminogen activator (tPA) is a thrombolytic agent.

127. The answer is d. *(Guyton, pp 428–429.)* The citrate ion has three anionic carboxylate groups that avidly chelate calcium and reduce the concentration of free calcium in blood. Because free calcium (Ca^{2+}) is required for multiple steps in both coagulation pathways, citrate is a useful anticoagulant in vitro. The citrate ion is rapidly metabolized; thus, blood anticoagulated with citrate can be infused into the body without untoward effects. Oxalate, another calcium-chelating anticoagulant, is toxic to cells.

128. The answer is d. *(Guyton, pp 428–429.)* An abnormally small number of platelets in the blood is called thrombocytopenia. Bleeding time is used to distinguish hemostatic abnormalities caused by a reduced number of platelets from those caused by coagulation defects. Hemostasis following blood vessel injury depends on (1) vascular spasm, (2) formation of a platelet plug, and (3) clot formation. The time for a small cut to stop bleeding depends on the concentration of platelets. Aspirin diminishes platelet aggregation by inhibiting cyclooxygenase, an enzyme required for generation of thromboxanes, which promote platelet aggregation.

129. The answer is c. *(Boron, pp 1197–1204. Guyton, pp 249–251, 960–962.)* Persistent fetal circulation (or persistent pulmonary hypertension) occurs when the normal reduction of pulmonary resistance does not occur at birth, resulting in a severe right to left shunt. In the womb, very little blood enters the lung. Forty percent of the blood entering the right atrium passes into the left atrium through the foramen ovale. The remaining blood is pumped into the pulmonary artery. However, almost all of this blood (90%) flows into the aorta through the ductus arteriosus. At birth, a rise in pulmonary resistance causes the foramen ovale and ductus arteriosus to close. If the pulmonary resistance is not decreased, the persistence of a significant right to left shunt prevents blood from being properly oxygenated, even when supplemental oxygen is administered.

130. The answer is d. (*Boron, pp 430–435. Guyton, pp 146–148, 247.*) Angiography in this patient revealed a 95% occlusion of the carotid artery. Turbulence, and consequently the bruit, was produced by the high velocity of blood within the stenotic area of the carotid artery. The widening of a vessel associated with aneurisms can also produce bruits but these are not relieved by endarterectomy. The likelihood of turbulence can be predicted from Reynolds number $\left(\dfrac{2v\rho}{\eta}\right)$ where

$$v = \text{velocity,}$$
$$\rho = \text{density,}$$
$$r = \text{radius and}$$
$$\eta = \text{viscosity}$$

131. The answer is b. (*Boron, pp 554–556. Guyton, pp 201–204.*) Angiotensin II is a powerful vasoconstrictor that is formed when renin is released from the kidney in response to a fall in blood pressure or vascular volume. Renin converts angiotensinogen to angiotensin I. Angiotensin II is formed from angiotensin I by an angiotensin-converting enzyme localized within the vasculature of the lung. All the other listed substances cause vasodilation.

132. The answer is b. (*Boron, pp 561–562. Guyton, p 192.*) A high intracranial pressure produces the Cushing reaction in which both sympathetic and parasympathetic input to the cardiovascular system increase. The parasympathetic stimulation of the heart causes the heart rate to decrease. The sympathetic stimulation to the blood vessels causes an extremely large increase in peripheral resistance. The sympathetic stimulation to the heart causes an increase in contractility, which, in turn, produces an increase in stroke volume. The Cushing reaction produces a rise in blood pressure, allowing the brain to be perfused despite high intracranial pressure (pressure as high as 300 to 400 mmHg).

133. The answer is d. *(Boron, pp 1252–1254.)* Exercise training decreases the resting heart rate. To maintain the same cardiac output with a lower heart rate, stroke volume is increased. Exercise training increases the aerobic capacity of an individual by increasing both the density of capillaries supplying the trained muscle and the concentration of mitochondria within the muscles. These changes allow the muscles to extract more oxygen from the blood perfusing them. At the same time, they permit a higher intensity of exercise during which a greater amount of oxygen can be used. Therefore, the maximum oxygen consumption (MVO_2) of trained individuals is above average.

134. The answer is b. *(Boron, pp 561–562, 582–585.)* Blood flow to the brain remains constant during exercise. To counteract the increased perfusion pressure that occurs during exercise, an autoregulatory process increases vascular resistance. The increase in mean blood pressure during exercise occurs despite a decrease in vascular resistance, because of the large increase in cardiac output. The decreased vascular resistance allows more blood to enter the exercising muscles during diastole, resulting in a lower diastolic pressure. Blood flow to the kidney is decreased in order to shunt blood to the heart and exercising muscles. Circulating blood volume decreases during exercise because of the increased capillary pressures within the exercising muscles and the accumulation of metabolites in the interstitial spaces, which produces an osmotic flow of water out of the capillaries.

135. The answer is e. *(Boron, pp 435–439.)* Pulse pressure is the difference between the systolic and diastolic pressure that occurs during the cardiac cycle. It is determined by the change in volume in the aorta during systole and the compliance of the aorta. A decrease in aortic compliance (that is, an increase in the stiffness of the aorta) will increase pulse pressure. When mean arterial pressure increases, the average volume of blood in the aorta is higher than normal. The increased volume decreases aortic compliance.

Assuming that the stroke volume remains normal, the decreased compliance will result in an increased pulse pressure. If heart rate increases, stroke volume and therefore pulse pressure will decrease. An increase in total peripheral resistance will prevent blood from flowing out of the aorta during systole and therefore decrease pulse pressure. In aortic stenosis, the rate at which blood is ejected from the ventricle is decreased. The decreased ejection rate provides time for blood to flow from the aorta to the periphery during systole. Therefore, the increase in aortic volume during systole and the pulse pressure are decreased.

136. The answer is b. *(Boron, pp 447–453, 477–481.)* The arterioles control the flow of blood to the various organs of the body. The resistance of the arterioles is controlled by the sympathetic nervous system and metabolites released by the organs. When the organs are very active (e.g., exercising skeletal muscle), the metabolites increase blood flow, even when the sympathetic stimulation of the arterioles is high. When metabolic production is low (e.g., nonexercising muscle), the amount of blood flowing into the organ is controlled by the sympathetic nervous system. The precapillary sphincters control the distribution of blood within an organ, supplying blood to cells that are more active and restricting blood flow to those that are less active. The arteries, postcapillary venules, and veins are not involved in regulation of blood flow through individual organs.

137. The answer is d. *(Boron, pp 475–476.)* Lymph flow is proportional to the amount of fluid filtered out of the capillaries. The amount of fluid filtered out of the capillaries depends on the Starling forces and capillary permeability. Increasing capillary oncotic pressure directly decreases filtration by increasing the hydrostatic (osmotic) force drawing water into the capillary. Increasing capillary pressure, capillary permeability, and interstitial protein concentration (oncotic pressure) all directly increase lymph flow. When venous pressure is increased, the capillary hydrostatic pressure is increased and, again, capillary filtration is increased. Lymph flow is approximately 2 to 3 L per day.

138. The answer is e. *(Boron, pp 585–590.)* Loss of blood causes blood pressure to fall. The baroreceptor reflex response to the fall in blood pressure causes arteriolar resistance to increase, further decreasing capillary

perfusing pressure. Because whole blood is lost, the concentration of circulating proteins remains normal and, therefore, the oncotic pressure remains
the same. The decreased capillary pressure and normal oncotic pressure
result in the transfer of fluid from the interstitium to the vascular bed,
decreasing the hematocrit. The increased arteriolar constriction lowers
blood flow to the kidney causing urine formation to decrease. Sympathetic
stimulation causes peripheral constriction and produces sweating, resulting in the classic sign of hemorrhage: cold, damp skin. The baroreceptor
reflex increases heart rate.

139. The answer is a. *(Boron, p 570. Guyton, pp 254–261.)* Anaphylactic
shock is characterized by a decreased peripheral resistance and a high cardiac output. The decrease in peripheral resistance is so great that mean
blood pressure falls below normal. Hypovolumic shock is caused by a
decrease in circulating blood volume and pressure. In both types of shock,
the baroreceptor reflex increases ventricular contractility and heart rate.
Also, in both types of shock, blood is shunted away from the kidney,
decreasing renal blood flow and glomerular filtration. As a result, plasma
creatinine levels rise.

140. The answer is e. *(Boron, pp 536–540.)* In some individuals the
baroreceptors can be activated by external mechanical deformation of the
carotid artery. The normal response of baroreceptor reflex activation is to
stimulate the vagal nerve in an attempt to slow heart rate and, therefore,
cardiac output and mean blood pressure. In some cases, emergency room
physicians will massage the neck to produce a baroreceptor reflex as a
means of slowing the heart rate. In this patient, turning his neck stimulated
the baroreceptor reflex, reducing blood flow to his head that caused lightheadedness. The baroreceptor reflex response to carotid sinus stimulation
will also decrease total peripheral resistance, venous tone, and ventricular
contractility. The reduction in venous tone will decrease central venous
pressure and, therefore, right atrial pressure.

141. The answer is b. *(Guyton, pp 170–174, Boron, pp 475–477.)* The primary function of the lymphatic vessels is to absorb the proteins that enter
the interstitial fluid from the systemic capillaries. Vascular and lymphatic
vessels share many characteristics: terminal arterials and lymphatics dis-
play vasomotor activity; both are involved in absorbing nutrients from the

GI tract, both have valves, and the capillary vessels in both systems are composed of endothelial cells.

142. The answer is b. *(Boron, p 1065.)* Pheochromocytoma is a tumor of the adrenal medulla characterized by an excessive release of catecholamines. Severe hypertension can result from the increase in heart rate and contractility (β-adrenergic activation by catecholamines) and vascular resistance (α-adrenergic activation). Blocking the α-adrenergic receptors will cause a decrease in TPR and a decrease in blood pressure.

143. The answer is a. *(Boron, pp 656–659. Guyton, pp 266, 390–391.)* Polycythemia vera is a disease in which an abnormally large number of red blood cells are produced. The large number of red blood cells causes an increase in blood viscosity by two or three times normal. Patients with polycythemia vera often have high blood pressure (because of increased blood volume) and cyanosis (because of increased oxygen extraction from blood flowing slowly through capillaries).

144–146. The answers are 144-a, 145-e, 146-c. *(Boron, pp 550–554.)* The diagram represents the cardiac and venous function curves that are often referred to as the Guyton curves. The cardiac function curves, which are similar to the familiar Starling curves, graph cardiac output as a function of central venous pressure. The cardiac function curves are shifted up and to the left by an increase in contractility and a decrease in afterload; they are shifted down and to the right by a decrease in contractility and an increase in afterload. The vascular function curves graph central venous pressure as a function of cardiac output. The graph is somewhat unusual in that the independent variable, cardiac output, is represented on the y axis. According to the vascular function curves, an increase in cardiac output causes a fall in central venous pressure. A decrease in blood volume or venous tone shifts the vascular function curves to the left; an increase in blood volume or venous tone shifts the vascular function curves to the right. The point at which the two curves intersect represents the central venous pressure and cardiac output of the cardiovascular system. An increase in total peripheral resistance (TPR) decreases the slope; a decrease in TPR increases the slope. An increase in TPR decreases the slope of the vascular function curve, and the increase in contractility shifts the cardiac function curve up and to the right. The new intersection of these curves is at point **A**. The shift from the resting state to point **E** represents an increase in vascular volume or venous tone without any change in TPR or ventricular contractility. This is consistent with a blood transfusion. The shift from the resting state to point **B** represents an increase in contractility with no change in TPR. This is consistent with the administration of a positive inotropic drug. When a person suddenly stands up, contractility and TPR increase, whereas venous compliance decreases (i.e., venous tone increases). When a person begins to exercise, there is an increase in contractility and a decrease in TPR and venous compliance.

Gastrointestinal Physiology

Questions

DIRECTIONS: Each question below contains five suggested responses. Select the **one best** response to each question.

147. A 27-year-old female comes to the emergency room because of a 2-day bout of profuse, watery diarrhea. Physical examination reveals dry lips and oropharynx. Laboratory values are normal except for a decreased serum K^+ (3.1 meq/L) and a decreased $Paco_2$ (18 mmHg). The patient is diagnosed with acute secretory diarrhea and dehydration, likely due to enterotoxigenic *Escherichia coli*. Which sodium reabsorptive pathway is inhibited by the enterotoxin?

a. Sodium-glucose-coupled cotransport
b. Electroneutral NaCl transport
c. Electrogenic sodium diffusion
d. Sodium-hydrogen countertransport
e. Sodium-bile salt cotransport

148. Which of the following statements about small intestinal motility is correct?

a. Contractile frequency is constant from duodenum to terminal ileum
b. Peristalsis is the major contractile pattern during feeding
c. Migrating motor complexes occur during the digestive period
d. Vagotomy abolishes contractile activity during the digestive period
e. Contractile activity is initiated in response to bowel wall distention

149. Which of the following statements about gastric emptying is correct?

a. Solids empty more rapidly than liquids
b. Vagotomy accelerates the emptying of solids
c. Indigestible food empties during the digestive period
d. Acidification of the antrum decreases gastric emptying
e. Vagotomy decreases accommodation of the proximal stomach

150. Vitamin B_{12} is absorbed primarily in which of the following organs?

a. Stomach
b. Duodenum
c. Jejunum
d. Ileum
e. Colon

151. Which of the following is the principal paracrine secretion involved in the inhibitory feedback regulation of gastric acid secretion?

a. Gastrin
b. Somatostatin
c. Histamine
d. Enterogastrone
e. Acetylcholine

152. Which of the following is the putative inhibitory neurotransmitter responsible for relaxation of gastrointestinal smooth muscle?

a. Dopamine
b. Vasoactive intestinal peptide
c. Somatostatin
d. Substance P
e. Acetylcholine

153. A 57-year-old man undergoes resection of the distal 100 cm of the terminal ileum as part of treatment for Crohn's disease. The patient likely will develop malabsorption of which of the following?

a. Iron
b. Folate
c. Lactose
d. Bile salts
e. Protein

154. A 42-year-old salesman presents with the chief complaint of intermittent midepigastric pain that is relieved by antacids or eating. Gastric analysis reveals that basal and maximal acid output exceed normal values. The gastric hypersecretion can be explained by an increase in the plasma concentration of which of the following?

a. Somatostatin
b. Histamine
c. Gastrin
d. Secretin
e. Enterogastrone

155. Which of the following statements best describes water and electrolyte absorption in the GI tract?

a. Most water and electrolytes come from ingested fluids
b. The small intestine and colon have similar absorptive capacities
c. Osmotic equilibration of chyme occurs in the stomach
d. The majority of absorption occurs in the jejunum
e. Water absorption is independent of Na^+ absorption

156. Hypokalemic metabolic acidosis can occur with excess fluid loss from which of the following organs?

a. Stomach
b. Ileum
c. Colon
d. Pancreas
e. Liver

157. Which of the following gastrointestinal motor activities is most affected by vagotomy?

a. Secondary esophageal peristalsis
b. Distention-induced intestinal segmentation
c. Orad stomach accommodation
d. Caudad stomach peristalsis
e. Migrating motor complexes

158. Which of the following hormones is involved in the initiation of the migrating motor complex?

a. Gastrin
b. Motilin
c. Secretin
d. Cholecystokinin
e. Enterogastrone

159. The rate of gastric emptying increases with an increase in which of the following?

a. Intragastric volume
b. Intraduodenal volume
c. Fat content of duodenum
d. Osmolality of duodenum
e. Acidity of duodenum

160. Basal acid output is increased by which of the following?

a. Acidification of the antrum
b. Administration of an H_2 receptor antagonist
c. Vagotomy
d. Alkalinization of the antrum
e. Acidification of the duodenum

161. Which of the following processes applies to the proximal stomach?

a. Accommodation
b. Peristalsis
c. Retropulsion
d. Segmentation
e. Trituration

162. After secretion of trypsinogen into the duodenum, the enzyme is converted into its active form, trypsin, by which of the following?

a. Enteropeptidase
b. Procarboxypeptidase
c. Pancreatic lipase
d. Chymotrypsin
e. An alkaline pH

163. Which of the following is the major mechanism for absorption of sodium from the small intestine?

a. Na^+-H^+ exchange
b. Cotransport with potassium
c. Electrogenic transport
d. Neutral NaCl absorption
e. Solvent drag

164. Pharmacological blockade of histamine H_2 receptors in the gastric mucosa

a. Inhibits both gastrin- and acetylcholine-mediated secretion of acid
b. Inhibits gastrin-induced but not meal-stimulated secretion of acid
c. Has no effect on either gastrin-induced or meal-stimulated secretion of acid
d. Prevents activation of adenyl cyclase by gastrin
e. Causes an increase in potassium transport by gastric parietal (oxyntic) cells

165. Removal of proximal segments of the small intestine results in a decrease in which of the following?

a. Basal acid output
b. Maximal acid output
c. Gastric emptying of liquids
d. Gastric emptying of solids
e. Pancreatic enzyme secretion

166. Dietary fat, after being processed, is extruded from the mucosal cells of the gastrointestinal tract into the lymphatic ducts in the form of

a. Monoglycerides
b. Diglycerides
c. Triglycerides
d. Chylomicrons
e. Free fatty acids

167. A 63-year-old female is diagnosed with an intractable duodenal ulcer. After consultation with a surgeon, it is recommended that she undergo a parietal cell vagotomy. Subsequently the patient experiences nausea and vomiting after ingestion of a mixed meal. Which of the following best explains her symptoms?

a. Increased gastric emptying of solids
b. Decreased gastric emptying of solids
c. Increased gastric emptying of liquids
d. Decreased gastric emptying of liquids
e. Increased emptying of liquids and solids

168. A 17-year-old male who is being treated with the macrolide antibiotic erythromycin complains of nausea, intestinal cramping, and diarrhea. The side effects are the result of the antibiotic binding to receptors on GI tract enteric nerves and smooth-muscle cells that recognize which gastrointestinal hormone?

a. Gastrin
b. Motilin
c. Secretin
d. Cholecystokinin
e. Enterogastrone

169. A 23-year-old woman complains of abdominal cramps and bloating that is relieved by defecation. Subsequent clinical evaluation reveals an increased maximal acid output, decreased serum calcium and iron concentrations, and microcytic anemia. Inflammation in which area of the GI tract would explain these findings?

a. Stomach
b. Duodenum
c. Jejunum
d. Ileum
e. Colon

170. Gastric emptying studies performed on a 49-year-old female reveal a time to one-half emptying of liquids of 18 min (normal <20 min) and a time to one-half emptying of solids to be 150 min (normal <120 min). Which of the following best explains the data?

a. Inflammation of the proximal small intestine
b. Surgical removal of the antrum
c. Pyloric stenosis
d. Decreased orad stomach compliance
e. Sectioning of the vagus nerves to the stomach

171. A 57-year-old female undergoes resection of the terminal ileum as part of treatment for her chronic inflammatory bowel disease. Removal of the terminal ileum will result in which of the following?

a. Increased bile acid concentration in the enterohepatic circulation
b. Decreased glucose absorption
c. Increased water content of the feces
d. Decreased fat absorption
e. Increased fat absorption

172. A 67-year-old male with a history of alcohol abuse presents to the emergency room with severe epigastric pain, hypotension, abdominal distension, and diarrhea with steatorrhea. Serum amylase and lipase are found to be greater than normal, leading to a diagnosis of pancreatitis. The steatorrhea can be accounted for by a decrease in the intraluminal concentration of which pancreatic enzyme?

a. Amylase
b. Trypsin
c. Chymotrypsin
d. Lipase
e. Colipase

173. A 42-year-old male is referred to a gastroenterologist for evaluation of refractory peptic ulcer disease. Subsequent endoscopic and laboratory data are suggestive of Zollinger-Ellison syndrome. The increased basal acid output and maximal acid output of the patient is best explained by an increase in plasma

a. Gastrin-releasing peptide concentrations
b. Secretin concentrations
c. Somatostatin concentrations
d. Gastrin concentrations
e. Histamine concentrations

174. Gas within the colon is primarily derived from which of the following sources?

a. CO_2 liberated by the interaction of HCO_3^- and H^+
b. Diffusion from the blood
c. Fermentation of undigested oligosaccharides by bacteria
d. Swallowed atmospheric air
e. Air pockets within foodstuffs

175. Removal of the pyloric sphincter is associated with which of the following?

a. A decrease in gastric compliance
b. An increase in maximal output of acid
c. An increase in basal output of acid
d. An increase in the rate of gastric emptying of solids
e. An increase in the serum gastrin level

176. Removal of the terminal ileum will result in which of the following?

a. A decrease in absorption of amino acids
b. An increase in the water content of the feces
c. An increase in the concentration of bile acid in the enterohepatic circulation
d. A decrease in the fat content of the feces
e. An increase in the absorption of iron

177. Vitamins synthesized by intestinal bacteria and absorbed in significant quantities include

a. Vitamin B_6
b. Vitamin K
c. Thiamine
d. Riboflavin
e. Folic acid

178. Which of the following statements about the colon is correct?

a. Absorption of Na^+ in the colon is under hormonal (aldosterone) control
b. Bile acids enhance absorption of water from the colon
c. Net absorption of HCO_3^- occurs in the colon
d. Net absorption of K^+ occurs in the colon
e. The luminal potential in the colon is positive

179. Contraction of the gallbladder is correctly described by which of the following statements?

a. It is inhibited by a fat-rich meal
b. It is inhibited by the presence of amino acids in the duodenum
c. It is stimulated by atropine
d. It occurs in response to cholecystokinin
e. It occurs simultaneously with the contraction of the sphincter of Oddi

180. Acidification of the duodenum will

a. Decrease pancreatic secretion of bicarbonate
b. Increase secretion of gastric acid
c. Decrease gastric emptying
d. Increase contraction of the gallbladder
e. Increase contraction of the sphincter of Oddi

181. Which of the following statements about small intestine crypt cells is correct?

a. They evidence well-developed microvilli
b. They are responsible for net NaCl and water absorption
c. They contain significant quantities of brush border hydrolases
d. They are responsible for net NaCl and water secretion
e. They demonstrate little or no proliferative activity

182. In contrast to secondary esophageal peristalsis, primary esophageal peristalsis is characterized by which of the following statements?

a. It does not involve relaxation of the lower esophageal sphincter
b. It involves only contraction of esophageal smooth muscle
c. It is not influenced by the intrinsic nervous system
d. It has an oropharyngeal phase
e. It involves only contraction of esophageal skeletal muscle

183. Absorption of fat-soluble vitamins requires

a. Intrinsic factor
b. Chymotrypsin
c. Pancreatic lipase
d. Pancreatic amylase
e. Secretin

184. Which of the following sugars is absorbed from the small intestine by facilitated diffusion?

a. Glucose
b. Galactose
c. Fructose
d. Sucrose
e. Lactose

185. Nearly all binding of cobalamin (vitamin B_{12}) to intrinsic factor occurs in which of the following organs?

a. Stomach
b. Duodenum
c. Jejunum
d. Ileum
e. Colon

186. Secondary esophageal peristalsis

a. Is preceded by an oral-pharyngeal phase of swallowing
b. Involves activation of medullary swallowing centers
c. Is accompanied by lower esophageal sphincter relaxation
d. Occurs in both the skeletal and smooth muscle portions of the esophagus
e. Is abolished by vagotomy

187. At concentrations present in the diet, which of the following vitamins is absorbed primarily by diffusion?

a. Vitamin C
b. Folate
c. Vitamin D
d. Niacin
e. Vitamin B_{12}

188. As compared to long-chain fatty acids, medium-chain fatty acids

a. Are also packaged as chylomicrons
b. Can be used as a source of calories in patients with malabsorptive disease
c. Are more abundant in the diet
d. Are less water-soluble
e. Are also returned to the circulation via the lymph

189. A 53-year-old male complains of a mild chronic cough and heartburn. Esophageal manometric and endoscopic evaluation reveal a hypotensive lower esophageal sphincter (LES) pressure and mild gastroesophageal reflux. Which of the following is the primary genesis of LES pressure in adults?

a. Tonic excitatory sympathetic nerve input to the smooth muscle
b. Tonic excitatory parasympathetic nerve input to the smooth muscle
c. Circulating gastrin
d. Myogenic properties of LES smooth muscle
e. Local production of nitric oxide by enteric nerves

190. A 42-year-old airline pilot presents to his family physician with a chief complaint of midepigastric pain that is relieved by antacids or eating. Endoscopic evaluation reveals the presence of a duodenal ulcer. Based on the diagnosis, which of the following also would be expected?

a. Decreased basal acid output
b. Increased maximal acid output
c. Decreased gastric emptying of liquids
d. Increased frequency of antral contractions
e. Decreased orad stomach compliance

191. A 26-year-old male presents to the emergency room with a 48-hour bout of diarrhea with steatorrhea. Which of the following could account for the appearance of excess fat in the stool?

a. Decreased bile salt pool size
b. Delayed gastric emptying
c. Decreased gastric acid secretion
d. Decreased secretion of intrinsic factor
e. Decreased gastric accommodation

192. A 43-year-old female presents with chief complaints of bulky and frequent diarrhea and weight loss. She experiences recurrent episodes of abdominal distension terminated by passage of stools. Laboratory data reveals a microcytic anemia, decreased serum calcium, and decreased serum albumin. After additional tests she is diagnosed with gluten-sensitive enteropathy. Her generalized decrease in intestinal absorption can be attributed to which of the following?

a. Decreased intestinal motility
b. Increased migrating motor complexes
c. Decreased intestinal surface area
d. Increased enterohepatic circulation of bile
e. Decreased gastric emptying

193. A 32-year-old woman presents to the emergency department with abdominal pain and diarrhea accompanied by steatorrhea. Gastric analysis reveals a basal acid output (12 mmol/h) greater than normal (<5 mmol/h). The steatorrhea is most likely due to which of the following?

a. Inactivation of pancreatic lipase due to low duodenal pH
b. Delayed gastric emptying
c. Decreased gastric acid secretion
d. Decreased secretion of intrinsic factor
e. Decreased pyloric sphincter tone

194. Severe inflammation of the ileum may be accompanied by which of the following?

a. Increased vitamin B_{12} absorption
b. Decreased bile acid pool size
c. Increased colon absorption of water
d. Decreased release of secretin
e. Increased absorption of dietary fats

195. Which one of the following statements about the process of vitamin B_{12} absorption is correct?

a. In humans, intrinsic factor is secreted from chief cells of the gastric gland
b. Vitamin B_{12} binds preferentially to intrinsic factor in the stomach
c. In adults, vitamin B_{12} absorption occurs along the length of the small intestine
d. Absorption may be reduced in a patient with pancreatic insufficiency
e. Absorption occurs via passive diffusion into the enterocyte

196. Patients may experience nausea and a sense of early satiety following which of the following procedures?

a. Surgical resection of the proximal small bowel
b. A vagotomy of the distal stomach
c. Surgical resection of the proximal stomach
d. Surgical removal of the gastric antrum
e. A vagotomy of the orad stomach

197. Which of the following is the origin of electrical slow wave activity in gastrointestinal tract smooth muscle?

a. The interstitial cells of Cajal
b. The smooth muscle of the circular muscle layer
c. The smooth muscle of the longitudinal muscle layer
d. The smooth muscle of the muscularis mucosa
e. The myenteric plexus

198. Which of the following statements is correct?

a. Pepsin is inactivated at a pH of 3 and below
b. Enterooxyntin is a small intestinal hormone inhibitory to gastric acid secretion
c. Gastric acid secretion is greatest during the cephalic phase of digestion
d. Somatostatin increases antral G cell gastrin release
e. Maximal acid output may be increased in a patient with duodenal ulcer disease

199. Which of the following is the major factor that protects the duodenal mucosa from damage by gastric acid?

a. Pancreatic bicarbonate secretion
b. The endogenous mucosal barrier of the duodenum
c. Duodenal bicarbonate secretion
d. Hepatic bicarbonate secretion
e. Bicarbonate contained in bile

200. Bicarbonate absorption from the upper small intestine is closely coupled with which of the following?

a. Na-glucose absorption
b. Neutral NaCl absorption
c. Na/H exchange
d. Electrogenic Na absorption
e. Na-vitamin B_{12} absorption

201. Which of the following statements about bile acids is correct?

a. Conjugation with glycine enhances passive absorption of bile acids
b. Bile acids constitute approximately 80% of the total solutes in bile
c. Deoxycholic acid and lithocholic acid are examples of primary bile acids
d. Bile acid synthesis is catalyzed by the microsomal enzyme 7α-hydroxylase
e. Bile acids are essentially water-insoluble

202. Withdrawal from chronic administration of an antisecretory compound is followed by rebound gastric acid hypersecretion. Which of the following drugs could account for the observed result?

a. A H_1 receptor antagonist
b. A proton pump inhibitor
c. A cholinergic receptor antagonist
d. An antacid
e. A CCKB receptor antagonist

203. The migrating motor complex in humans

a. Occurs only in the small intestine
b. Requires an intact intrinsic nervous system for coordinated propagation
c. Is the result of food-mediated distension of the small intestine
d. Mixes intestinal contents with bile and the digestive enzymes
e. Is correlated with periodic increases in plasma gastrin levels

204. The delivery of chyme into the proximal small intestine will

a. Increase gastric acid secretion
b. Decrease pancreatic bicarbonate secretion
c. Increase gastric emptying of solids
d. Decrease circulating CCK levels
e. Increase small intestine segmentation

205. A 61-year-old male presents to his family physician with the chief complaint of frequent diarrhea accompanied by weight loss. He reports a tendency to bruise easily and laboratory data reveal a prothrombin time of 19 s (normal = 11 to 14 s). The bruising and prolonged prothrombin time can be explained by a decrease in which of the following vitamins?

a. Vitamin A
b. Vitamin C
c. Vitamin D
d. Vitamin E
e. Vitamin K

206. A 49-year-old female is referred to surgery for removal of a tumor from the fundic region of the stomach. Resection of the fundus will likely result in which of the following outcomes?

a. A decrease in the contractile frequency of the stomach
b. An increase in the gastric emptying rate of liquids
c. A decrease in the gastric emptying of solids
d. An increase in maximal acid output
e. A decreased gastrin release in response to ingestion of a meal

207. An 18-year-old college student reports that she experiences severe abdominal bloating and diarrhea within 1 hour of consuming dairy products. A subsequent H_2-breath test is abnormal. The diarrhea and bloating can be explained by which of the following?

a. A deficiency in the brush border enzyme lactase
b. Carbohydrate-induced secretory diarrhea
c. Decreased intestinal surface area
d. Decreased carbohydrate absorption
e. A decrease in exocrine pancreatic secretion

208. A 31-year-old male presents to the emergency room with the symptoms of heartburn and difficulty swallowing. Esophageal manometry reveals an inflammed esophageal mucosa and a hypotensive lower esophageal sphincter. A diagnosis of gastroesophageal reflux disease is made and the patient is subsequently treated with an H_2-receptor antagonist. Normally, reflux of gastric acid into the esophagus

a. Initiates primary esophageal peristalsis
b. Inhibits gastric acid secretion
c. Initiates secondary esophageal peristalsis
d. Inhibits esophageal bicarbonate secretion
e. Inhibits gastric motility

209. A 42-year-old obese female presents to the emergency department with right upper quadrant pain, nausea, and vomiting. The pain is not related to food intake and lasts for several hours before resolving slowly. Ultrasound and HIDA scan images are suggestive of gallstones with cystic duct obstruction. Which of the following is the primary physiological stimulus of gallbladder contraction in the digestive period?

a. Acid-induced release of secretin from the small intestine
b. Fat-induced release of cholecystokinin from the small intestine
c. Calorie-induced release of enterogastrone from the small intestine
d. Distension-induced release of glucagon from the small intestine
e. Amino acid–induced release of motilin from the small intestine

210. Which of the following statements best describes water and electrolyte absorption in the gastrointestinal tract?

a. Most water and electrolytes derive from the oral intake of fluids
b. The small and large intestines have similar absorptive capacities
c. Net secretion of potassium occurs from the ileum
d. Osmotic equilibration of chyme occurs in the duodenum
e. Cholera toxin inhibits sodium-coupled nutrient transport

211. The paracrine secretion responsible for inhibiting gastric acid secretion is which of the following?

a. Histamine
b. Enterogastrone
c. Somatostatin
d. Pepsin
e. Enterooxyntin

212. A medical student presents to the emergency room with a 2-day history of severe vomiting and orthostatic hypotension. What kind of metabolic abnormalities are most likely in this patient?

a. Hypokalemia, hypochloremia, and metabolic acidosis
b. Hyperkalemia, hyperchloremia, and metabolic alkalosis
c. Normal serum electrolytes and metabolic acidosis
d. Normal serum electrolytes and metabolic alkalosis
e. Hypokalemic, hypochloremic, metabolic alkalosis

213. The metabolic effects of insulin include which of the following?

a. Decreased glucose utilization
b. Decreased lipolysis
c. Increased proteolysis
d. Increased gluconeogenesis
e. Increased ketogenesis

214. Which of the following statements about bile acids is correct?

a. They are essentially water-insoluble
b. The majority of bile acids is absorbed by passive diffusion
c. Glycine conjugates are more soluble than taurine conjugates
d. The amount lost in the stool each day represents the daily loss of cholesterol
e. The bile acid–dependent fraction of bile is stimulated by the hormone secretin

215. In contrast to secretory diarrhea, osmotic diarrhea

a. Is characterized by an increase in stool osmolarity
b. Is the result of increased crypt cell secretion
c. Is the result of decreased electroneutral sodium absorption
d. Is caused by bacterial toxins
e. Occurs only in the colon

216. The transport protein responsible for entry of glucose into the intestinal enterocyte is called

a. Glut-2
b. Glut-5
c. SGLT1
d. SGLT2
e. SGLT5

217. Short-chain fatty acid absorption occurs almost exclusively from which of the following organs?

a. Stomach
b. Duodenum
c. Jejunum
d. Ileum
e. Colon

218. Which of the following statements about medium-chain fatty acids is correct?

a. They are more water-soluble than long-chain fatty acids
b. Within the enterocyte, they are used for triglyceride resynthesis
c. They are packaged into chylomicrons
d. They are transported in the lymph
e. They require emulsification prior to enterocyte uptake

Gastrointestinal Physiology

Answers

147. The answer is b. (*Boron, pp 933–940.*) Diarrhea is defined as the excretion of 200 g or more of water in the stools of an adult during a 24-h period. Although sodium is absorbed from the small intestine by several mechanisms, bacterial toxins specifically inhibit neutral NaCl absorption. In addition, the toxins augment diarrhea by increasing salt and water secretion by intestinal crypt cells. Oral rehydration involves utilizing the sodium-glucose-coupled cotransport pathway.

148. The answer is e. (*Boron, pp 888–890. Guyton, pp 723–724, 733–734.*) Segmentation, the primary motility pattern of the digestive period in humans, is defined as irregular and uncoordinated contraction of the circular muscle layer. This pattern, which develops in response to intestinal wall distention, is determined by activation of preprogrammed neural circuits within the myenteric plexus. The contractile frequency of the small intestine decreases in an aboral direction. The contractions, which are caused by underlying changes in smooth-muscle electrical activity called electrical slow waves, decrease from approximately 11 per minute in the duodenum to approximately 6 to 7 per minute in the distal ileum. Elimination of extrinsic input to the bowel wall has little functional effect on bowel motility during the digestive period. Segmentation develops immediately upon the delivery of food into the small intestine and is accompanied by abolishment of the migrating motor complexes characteristic of the interdigestive period.

149. The answer is e. (*Boron, pp 906–907. Guyton, pp 730–733.*) Distention of the orad stomach elicits an inhibitory vago-vagal accommodation reflex that controls intragastric pressure and the emptying of liquids. Removal of inhibitory vagal input leads to decreased gastric accommodation and increased emptying of liquid. Distention of the caudad stomach elicits an excitatory vago-vagal reflex that results in the trituration of solid food in particles 1 mm and smaller. Because solids must be liquefied prior to emptying from the stomach, the gastric emptying of liquids begins before the emptying of solids. The actual rate of emptying depends upon neural (enterogastric reflex) and hormonal (enterogastrone) inhibitory feedback from the proximal small bowel. Undigested food residue empties during the interdigestive period in concert with the development of migrating motor complexes.

150. The answer is d. *(Boron, pp 969–971. Guyton, pp 386–389, 811.)* Vitamin B_{12} (cobalamin) is absorbed primarily by the enterocysts of the distal ileum. Efficient absorption requires intrinsic factor, a glycoprotein secreted by the parietal cells of the gastric mucosa. The vitamin B_{12}-intrinsic factor complex is emptied from the stomach and propelled along the small intestine to the terminal ileum, where specific transporters located on the enterocyte microvilli bind the vitamin B_{12}-intrinsic factor complex. Binding requires calcium and is optimal at pH 6.6. Absorption is an active transport process.

151. The answer is b. *(Boron, pp 885–889. Guyton, pp 742–746.)* Somatostatin, located within the SS cells of the gastric antral mucosa, is the principal paracrine secretion involved in the inhibitory feedback of gastric acid secretion. Somatostatin is released in response to an increase in hydrogen ions. In humans, gastric acid secretion by the parietal cell occurs in response to excitatory neural (acetylcholine), hormonal (gastrin), and paracrine (histamine) stimuli. Inhibitory feedback regulation of acid output also involves neural (enterogastric reflex), hormonal (enterogastrone), and paracrine (somatostatin) influences.

152. The answer is b. *(Boron, pp 885. Guyton, pp 720–722.)* Important inhibitory neurotransmitters in the gastrointestinal tract include vasoactive intestinal peptide and nitric oxide. Relaxation of gastrointestinal smooth muscle occurs following activation of nonadrenergic, noncholinergic (NANC) enteric nerve fibers. Acetylcholine, substance P, and dopamine are excitatory neurotransmitters. Somatostatin is a paracrine secretory product with multiple effects on gastrointestinal function.

153. The answer is d. *(Boron, pp 960–964, 969–971.)* Removal of the terminal ileum can lead to diarrhea and steatorrea. The terminal ileum contains specialized cells responsible for the absorption of primary and secondary bile salts by active transport. Bile salts are necessary for adequate digestion and absorption of fat. In the absence of the terminal ileum there will be an increase in the amounts of bile acids and fatty acids delivered to the colon. Fats and bile salts in the colon increase the water content of the feces by promoting the influx (secretion) of water into the lumen of the colon.

154. The answer is c. *(Boron, pp 894–901.)* Increases in basal and maximal acid output are suggestive of inflammation of the proximal small intestine. Intestinal receptors monitor the composition of chyme and elicit feedback mechanisms that regulate gastric acid secretion and gastric emptying. Absence of feedback leads to an increased presence of excitatory mediators of gastric function. Gastrin is the primary stimulus of meal-induced acid secretion. Somatostatin (paracrine), secretin (endocrine), and enterogastrone (endocrine) inhibit gastric acid secretion. Histamine is an excitatory paracrine mediator of acid secretion.

155. The answer is d. *(Boron, pp 931–946. Guyton, pp 758–760.)* Most water and electrolyte absorption occurs in the jejunum, with the duodenum serving primarily as the site of osmotic equilibration of chyme. Water absorption is passive and occurs as the direct result of active sodium absorption. The small intestine and colon absorb approximately 9 to 12 L of fluid per 24-h period, most of which comes from gastrointestinal secretions. In contrast to the small intestine, the colon has a limited capacity to absorb water (approximately 3 to 6 L per day).

156. The answer is c. *(Boron, pp 890–892. Guyton, p 762.)* Loss of gastric juice results in hypokalemic, metabolic alkalosis. Excessive loss of fluid from the gastrointestinal tract can lead to dehydration and, depending on the origin of the fluid loss, electrolyte and acid-base disturbances. The hydrogen ion and potassium ion concentration of gastric juice exceeds that of the plasma. As a result, excess fluid loss leads to metabolic alkalosis accompanied by hypokalemia. Because the pancreas, liver, ileum, and colon secrete bicarbonate, excessive loss leads to metabolic acidosis. In addition, the colon secretes potassium. Thus, the acidosis is accompanied by hypokalemia.

157. The answer is c. *(Boron, p 906. Guyton, pp 598–610.)* Orad stomach accommodation depends exclusively on an intact vago-vagal reflex. Vagal innervation of the gastrointestinal tract extends from the esophagus to the level of the transverse colon. Preganglionic fibers from cell bodies in the medulla synapse with ganglion cells located in the enteric nervous system.

Distention-induced contraction of gastrointestinal smooth muscle develops as the result of long (vago-vagal) and local (enteric nerves) reflexes. The importance of long versus local reflex pathways varies along the gut. Secondary esophageal peristalsis, intestinal segmentation, and migrating motor complexes are unaffected by vagotomy, whereas caudad stomach peristalsis is decreased but not abolished by vagotomy.

158. The answer is b. (*Boron, pp 885, 890. Guyton, p 610.*) Motilin is released during the interdigestive period and is believed to be involved in the initiation of the migrating motor complex. The factors responsible for release are unknown. All other gastrointestinal hormones are released during the digestive period and coordinate motor and secretory activities.

159. The answer is a. (*Boron, pp 906–907.*) The initial rate of emptying varies directly with the volume of the meal ingested. Gastric emptying is influenced by the intragastric volume and by the physical and chemical composition of the chyme in the small intestine. Increasing the volume, fat content, acidity, or osmolarity of the lumen of the small intestine elicits inhibitory neural (enterogastric reflex) and hormonal (enterogastrone) feedback mechanisms.

160. The answer is d. (*Boron, pp 899–901. Guyton, pp 730–733.*) Alkalinization of the antrum releases the gastrin-containing cells from the inhibitory influences of somatostatin and increases acid secretion. Acidification of the antrum promotes the release of somatostatin, a paracrine secretion that inhibits gastrin release. Decreased gastrin release reduces the acid output of the stomach. Acidification of the duodenum elicits inhibitory neural (enterogastric) and hormonal (enterogastrone) reflexes that also inhibit acid output. Administration of a histamine antagonist reduces acid secretion by decreasing the stimulatory effect of histamine.

161. The answer is a. (*Boron, pp 906–907.*) Increases in intragastric volume normally are not associated with large increases in intragastric pressure because of distention-mediated activation of a vago-vagal inhibitory reflex, the accommodation reflex. The reflex is a property of the proximal stomach only and counterbalances the stretch-induced myogenic contraction of the gastric smooth muscle. Peristalsis, trituration (grinding), and retropulsion (mixing) are terms referring to the contractile activity and functions of the distal stomach. Segmentation is the primary contractile pattern of the small intestine during the digestive period.

162. The answer is a. *(Boron, p 924. Guyton, p 746.)* Liberation of the enzyme enteropeptidase (enterokinase) from the duodenal mucosal cells causes the inactive trypsinogen to be converted to the active form, trypsin. Enteropeptidase contains 41% polysaccharide. It is this high level of polysaccharide that protects enteropeptidase from digestion. Trypsin is responsible for the conversion of chymotrypsinogens and other proenzymes into their active forms.

163. The answer is d. *(Boron, pp 931–946. Guyton, pp 758–760.)* Although multiple pathways exist for the absorption of Na^+, neutral absorption is the major mechanism. Absorption of sodium is the primary absorptive event in the small intestine. Absorption of Na^+ is necessary for absorption of water and other electrolytes. Neutral absorption may occur in two ways: Na^+ cotransported with Cl^- or in exchange for H^+ ions.

164. The answer is a. *(Boron, pp 894–899. Guyton, 744–746.)* Histamine (H_2) receptor antagonists inhibit both gastrin-induced and vagal-mediated secretion of acid. Secretion of acid by gastric parietal (oxyntic) cells involves stimulation of adenyl cyclase and cyclic AMP–mediated stimulation of the active transport of chloride and potassium-hydrogen ion exchange. Neither gastrin nor vagal stimulation activates adenyl cyclase directly; both depend on concomitant release of histamine and histamine-induced activation of adenyl cyclase.

165. The answer is e. *(Boron, pp 898–899, 921–923. Guyton, pp 732–733, 745–748.)* Inflammation or removal of the upper small intestine leads to a decrease in pancreatic and hepatobiliary function. The proximal small intestine contains a number of "receptors" that monitor the physical (volume) and chemical (pH, fat content, caloric density, osmolality) composition of the chyme emptied from the stomach. Stimulation of these receptors releases hormones and activates neural reflexes that initiate pancreatic enzyme and bicarbonate secretion, stimulate gallbladder emptying, and provide feedback for inhibitory regulation of gastric function (enterogastrone, enterogastric reflex). Removal of these reflexes decreases pancreatic secretion and gallbladder emptying and increases gastric emptying and acid output.

166. The answer is d. (*Boron, pp 965–967. Guyton, pp 756–758.*) Long-chain fatty acids are extruded from enterocytes in the form of chylomicrons into the lymphatic system. Triglycerides are hydrolyzed to monoglycerides and taken into mucosal cells. If the fatty acids are short chains (less than 10 to 12 carbon atoms), they are extruded in the form of free fatty acids into the portal blood. Chylomicrons represent triglycerides and esters of cholesterol that have been invested in the intestinal mucosa with a coating of phospholipid, protein, and cholesterol.

167. The answer is b. (*Boron, pp 894–901, 906–907.*) The vagus nerve is the primary neural mediator of gastric function. Activation of distension-mediated vago-vagal reflexes in response to the presence of food in the stomach will (a) increase gastric compliance (accommodation reflex) and promote gastric retention of food, (b) increase the strength of antral peristaltic contractions necessary for trituration of solids, and (c) increase gastric acid secretion. Sectioning of the vagus nerve fibers to the antral region of the stomach will decrease the strength of contractions thereby prolonging the emptying of solids. The emptying of liquids will be unaffected.

168. The answer is b. (*Boron, pp 885, 890.*) Motilin is the gastrointestinal peptide hormone associated with the initiation of migrating motor complexes during the interdigestive period. The hormone stimulates increased contractions by a direct action on smooth muscle and by activation of excitatory enteric nerves. Erythromycin belongs to the group of macrolide antibiotics and also shows an ability to excite motilin-like receptors on enteric nerves and smooth muscle. As a result, a common side effect of the antibiotic is abdominal cramping and diarrhea.

169. The answer is b. (*Boron, pp 967–974. Guyton, pp 758–761.*) Inflammation of the duodenum may lead to increased acid output, hypocalcemia, and microcytic anemia. Increased basal and maximal acid outputs may result from excessive stimulation of the parietal cell (e.g., hypergastrinemia) or reduced inhibitory feedback (i.e., reduced effect of enterogastrone and the enterogastric reflex). The latter may occur when the proximal small intestine is inflamed. Although calcium is absorbed along the entire length of the small intestine, it is absorbed primarily in the duodenum. Similarly, iron is absorbed primarily in the duodenum. Microcytic anemia is the result of reduced stores of iron.

170. The answer is c. *(Boron, pp 906–907.)* The emptying of solids from the stomach is determined by the strength of antral peristaltic contractions and the resistance offered by the pyloric sphincter. Either a decrease in the amplitude of the antral contractions or an increase in sphincter resistance will delay the emptying of solids from the stomach. Liquid emptying is regulated by the proximal stomach and is primarily a function of the difference between the intragastric pressure and the intraduodenal pressure.

171. The answer is c. *(Boron, 960–964, 969–971.)* Removal of the terminal ileum can lead to diarrhea and steatorrhea. The terminal ileum contains specialized cells responsible for the absorption of primary and secondary bile salts by active transport. Bile salts are necessary for adequate digestion and absorption of fat. In the absence of the terminal ileum there will be an increase in the amounts of bile acids and fatty acids delivered to the colon. Fats and bile salts in the colon increase the water content of the feces by promoting the influx (secretion) of water into the lumen of the colon.

172. The answer is d. *(Boron, pp 918–924, 963–965.)* The process of fat digestion begins in the stomach and is completed in the proximal small intestine, predominately by enzymes synthesized and secreted by the pancreatic acinar cells. The major lipolytic pancreatic enzyme is the carboxylic esterase, known as lipase. Full activity requires the protein cofactor colipase, as well as an alkaline pH, bile salts, and fatty acids.

173. The answer is d. *(Boron, pp 894–901.)* Zollinger-Ellison patients have a pancreatic acinar cell adenoma (gastrinoma) characterized by the synthesis and secretion of large amounts of gastrin. Unlike gastrin released from the antrum in response to normal physiological stimuli, the pancreatic release of gastrin from the pancreas is not under physiological control, i.e., intestinal feedback and gastric pH.

174. The answer is c. *(Guyton, pp 769–770.)* Gas within the colon is derived primarily from fermentation of undigested material by intestinal bacteria to produce CO_2, H_2, and methane. The digestive tract normally contains about 150 to 200 mL of gas, most of which is in the colon (100 to 150 mL). Most of the gas in the stomach is derived from air swallowed during eating or in periods of anxiety. Gas is produced in the small intestine by interaction of gastric acid and bicarbonate in the intestinal and pancreatic secretions but does not accumulate because it is either reabsorbed or quickly passed into the colon. The amount of gas varies markedly from one person to another and is influenced by diet; for example, ingestion of large amounts of beans, which contain indigestible carbohydrates in their hulls, will increase gas formation by intestinal bacteria. Diffusion of gas from the blood to the intestinal lumen is responsible for the N_2 present in intestinal gas and is influenced by the atmospheric pressure.

175. The answer is d. (*Boron, pp 899–901, 906–907. Guyton, pp 730–733.*) Removal of the pyloric sphincter will increase the rate of gastric emptying because the resistance to flow of large particles will be removed. The distal stomach, which includes the antrum and the pyloric sphincter, is involved in the regulation of the gastric emptying of solids and in the regulation of gastric acid secretion. Antral peristaltic contractions promote the trituration of solids. The pyloric sphincter serves to limit the flow of solids out of the stomach until the particles are of a small enough size to be suspended in the liquid component of the meal. Secretion of acid will be decreased because of the loss of gastrin, which is normally secreted by the G cells of the antrum. Gastric compliance is a property of the proximal stomach.

176. The answer is b. (*Boron, 960–964, 969–971. Guyton, pp 750–751.*) Removal of the terminal ileum can lead to diarrhea and steatorrhea. The terminal ileum contains specialized cells responsible for the absorption of primary and secondary bile salts by active transport. Bile salts are necessary for adequate digestion and absorption of fat. In the absence of the terminal ileum there will be an increase in the amounts of bile acids and fatty acids delivered to the colon. Fats and bile salts in the colon increase the water content of the feces by promoting the influx (secretion) of water into the lumen of the colon. Amino acids are absorbed in the jejunum. Iron is primarily absorbed in the duodenum.

177. The answer is e. (*Boron, pp 967–969. Guyton, pp 967–969.*) Folic acid is both produced in the intestine and absorbed from the intestine. In humans, several vitamins, including vitamin K, several of the B complex, and folic acid, are synthesized by intestinal bacteria. However, only folic acid is absorbed by the host. Dietary intake of the other vitamins is necessary.

178. The answer is a. *(Boron, pp 931–946. Guyton, pp 758–763.)* Both the absorption of Na⁺ and secretion of K⁺ from the colon are affected by changes in circulating levels of aldosterone. The major route of absorption of sodium in the colon is electrogenic transport. Because of the "tight" nature of the tight junctions that connect cells in the colon, a relatively large potential difference exists between the mucosal (negative) and serosal (positive) surfaces of the absorptive cells. This electrical difference favors the net secretion of K⁺ into the lumen. Secretion of HCO_3^- occurs in exchange for absorption of Cl⁻. No counterbalancing cation exchange pumps are present in the colon.

179. The answer is d. *(Boron, pp 992–993. Guyton, pp 749–750.)* Cholecystokinin is released from the upper small intestine in response to partially hydrolyzed dietary lipids and proteins and promotes gallbladder emptying. Gallbladder contraction and sphincter of Oddi relaxation are necessary for delivery of bile into the duodenum. These muscular actions are under both hormonal and neural control. Cholecystokinin contracts gallbladder smooth muscle by a direct action on the muscle and through activation of vagal afferent fibers leading to a vago-vagal reflex. Relaxation of sphincter of Oddi smooth muscle occurs via activation of inhibitory enteric nerves. Vagal stimulation, which is cholinergically mediated and blocked by atropine, also promotes gallbladder contraction.

180. The answer is c. *(Boron, pp 899–901, 921–924. Guyton, pp 732–733.)* Acidification of the upper small intestine results in the inhibitory feedback regulation of gastric function. Secretin is released from the small intestine primarily in response to an increased delivery of hydrogen ions. Secretin is the primary stimulus for pancreatic secretion of water and bicarbonate. In addition secretin may serve as an enterogastrone, that is, a hormone involved in the inhibitory feedback regulation of gastric function. Cholecystokinin (CCK) is the hormone responsible for contraction of the gallbladder and relaxation of the sphincter of Oddi.

181. The answer is d. *(Boron, pp 931–933. Guyton, pp 752–753.)* Intestinal crypt cells are characterized by the transport of chloride and water into the intestinal lumen. Secretion of chloride across the apical cell membrane is believed to involve the cystic fibrosis transmembrane receptor (CFTR) chloride channel. Crypt cells are the proliferative cells of the intestinal mucosa. As crypt cells migrate up the villus axis, they undergo significant morphological and biochemical differentiation. They change from short, cuboidal cells with minimal microvilli and few apical membrane transporters or brush border hydrolases into mature villus tip cells prepared for the role of nutrient, water, and electrolyte absorption.

182. The answer is d. (*Boron, pp 886–887. Guyton, pp 728–730.*) Primary peristalsis involves not only esophageal peristalsis and relaxation of the lower esophageal sphincter (LES), but also the oral-pharyngeal phase of swallowing. The term primary esophageal peristalsis denotes that swallowing has been elicited as a consequence of activation of the "swallowing centers" in the medulla (nucleus ambiguus, dorsal motor X). Secondary esophageal peristalsis is a localized esophageal response to irritation or distention that results in a peristaltic contraction and relaxation of the LES. Both primary and secondary esophageal peristalsis require an intact intrinsic nervous system.

183. The answer is c. (*Boron, pp 918–919, 963.*) Absorption of the fat-soluble vitamins (A, D, E, and K) is diminished if there is a lack of pancreatic lipase. Lipase is required to produce monoglycerides that, in combination with bile salts, make it possible to bring the fat-soluble vitamins close to the mucosal cell surface for absorption. With the exception of vitamin B_{12}, which is absorbed bound to intrinsic factor in the ileum, vitamins are absorbed chiefly in the upper small intestine.

184. The answer is c. (*Boron, pp 947–953. Guyton, pp 761–762.*) Facilitated diffusion is the major transport route for fructose. The duodenum and jejunum are the principal sites of carbohydrate absorption in humans. Digestion of carbohydrates is accomplished by amylase and brush border enzymes and results in a mixture of glucose, fructose, and galactose. A common sodium-dependent secondary active transporter absorbs glucose and galactose. Sucrose and lactose are disaccharides that break down into glucose and fructose, and glucose and galactose, respectively.

185. The answer is b. (*Boron, pp 969–970.*) Although intrinsic factor is secreted by the oxyntic cells of the gastric mucosa, binding to cobalamin occurs in the duodenum. Cobalamin, also known as vitamin B_{12}, is synthesized only by microorganisms and, in the human diet, is provided almost entirely from animal products. Gastric digestion of food liberates cobalamin where, at low pH, it binds primarily to the R protein–type binder, haptocorrin, derived primarily from salivary secretions. In the duodenum, pancreatic proteases release cobalamin from the haptocorrin but have no effect on intrinsic factor derived from parietal cells. Cobalamin rapidly complexes with intrinsic factor and is transported along the gut to the distal 60 cm of the ileum, where specific receptors located on the villus tip cells bind the cobalamin-intrinsic factor complex.

186. The answer is c. *(Boron, pp 886–888. Guyton, pp 886–887.)* The term secondary esophageal peristalsis describes esophageal peristalsis and lower esophageal relaxation associated with distension or irritation of the smooth-muscle portion of the esophageal body. The event is limited to the smooth-muscle component of the esophagus and is the result of activation of enteric nerves. Initiation of secondary peristalsis does not involve extrinsic neural reflexes and, thus, is not accompanied by the oral-pharyngeal phase of swallowing.

187. The answer is c. *(Boron, pp 967–972. Guyton, pp 904–906.)* Absorption of vitamin D increases linearly as the intraluminal concentration increases, suggesting absorption by a nonsaturable passive-diffusion mechanism. The term vitamin D refers to a family of essentially water-insoluble compounds involved primarily in the regulation of calcium homeostasis. Water-soluble vitamins, including vitamin C, folate, niacin, and vitamin B_{12}, are a diverse group of organic compounds that are essential for normal growth and development. At the low concentrations present in the diet (1 to 100 nM), transport of the vitamins across the brush border occurs by specialized mechanisms, such as membrane carriers, active transport systems, and membrane-binding proteins and receptors, specific for a particular vitamin.

188. The answer is b. *(Boron, pp 960–967.)* Medium-chain triglycerides (MCTs) are readily absorbed from the small intestine and can be used as a source of calories in patients with a wide variety of GI diseases resulting in malabsorption. MCTs are fatty acids of 6 to 12 carbon chain lengths that are present in small amounts in the normal diet. They are hydrolyzed by lipases more rapidly than long-chain fatty acids and are much more water-soluble than long-chain triglycerides. MCTs are not utilized for resynthesis of triglycerides and therefore are not packaged into chylomicrons. Instead, they are released directly into the portal blood.

189. The answer is d. *(Boron, pp 886–888.)* The lower esophageal sphincter is a high-pressure zone that exists between the esophageal body and the gastric fundus. The high pressure limits reflux of gastric contents into the esophageal body. Although excitatory vagal input contributes to the high-pressure zone, the principal determinant is intrinsic (myogenic) properties of the circular smooth muscle of the sphincter. Excess acid in the esophagus creates the pain sensation referred to as heartburn.

190. The answer is b. *(Boron, pp 894–901, 906–907.)* Inflammation of the proximal small intestine results in a decrease in the feedback regulation of gastric function by reducing the input of the enterogastric reflex and enterogastrone to gastric emptying and gastric acid secretion. Absent inhibitory input, basal and maximal acid output are increased, and the gastric emptying of liquids and solids is increased.

191. The answer is a. *(Boron, pp 960–964, 969–971.)* Steatorrhea is defined as excess loss of fat in the stool. Numerous pathophysiological situations can cause the loss of excess fat in the stool including a decrease in bile acid pool size, inactivation or decreased intraluminal concentration of pancreatic lipase in the small intestine, and decreased intestinal absorptive surface area. A decrease in bile acid pool size results in an increased delivery of fats into the colon, which in turn inhibits fat absorption and promotes water secretion.

192. The answer is c. *(Boron, p 948.)* Gluten-sensitivity enteropathy is characterized by an autoimmune-induced decrease in the absorptive surface area of the small intestine. In addition to a decrease in the area available for absorption of nutrients, minerals, electrolytes and water, the membrane transporters of the remaining villous tip cells are impaired or absent.

193. The answer is a. *(Boron, pp 918–924, 963–964.)* The process of fat digestion begins in the stomach and is completed in the proximal small intestine, predominately by enzymes synthesized and secreted by the pancreatic acinar cells. The major lipolytic pancreatic enzyme is the carboxylic esterase, known as lipase. Full activity requires the protein cofactor colipase, bile salts, fatty acids, as well as an alkaline pH. Excess delivery of acid into the proximal small intestine leads to reduced lipolytic activity.

194. The answer is b. *(Boron, pp 963–971. Guyton, pp 766–767.)* Individuals with inflammatory disease of the ileum have decreased bile acid pool size due to decreased bile acid reabsorption. This results in reduced absorption of dietary triglycerides and fat-soluble vitamins, including vitamin K. The efficient absorption of dietary fats requires the presence of critical concentrations of primary and secondary bile salts (1 to 5 mmol/L). Because the absolute amount of bile acids available for fat digestion during a meal (the bile acid pool size) is generally less than the amounts required for complete digestion and absorption, bile acids must be recirculated via the enterohepatic circulation. Conservation of bile acids during a meal is highly efficient and occurs primarily from the distal ileum via sodium-dependent, secondary active transport. The increased delivery of dietary fat and bile acids into the colon decreases colonic absorption of water. The loss of bile salts in the stool cannot be fully compensated for by increased hepatic synthesis, and, thus, there is a resultant decrease in bile acid pool size.

195. The answer is d. *(Boron, pp 969–971, 907.)* Patients with pancreatic insufficiency, as well as patients with Crohn's disease, bacterial overgrowth, or who have undergone ileal resection, may exhibit vitamin B_{12} deficiency. Cobalamin, also known as vitamin B_{12}, is an essential vitamin found in such foods as liver, fish, and dairy products. Absorption of cobalamin occurs exclusively from the ileum, where specific receptors on ileal enterocytes bind a complex of cobalamin and intrinsic factor. Although intrinsic factor is secreted by gastric parietal cells, binding of the vitamin to intrinsic factor occurs primarily in the proximal small intestine. The acidic environment of the gastric lumen favors the binding of cobalamin to R protein–type binding proteins that originate from salivary and gastric secretions. Pancreatic proteases in the small intestine degrade the R proteins, and the rise in pH favors rapid and complete transfer of the vitamin to intrinsic factor.

196. The answer is b. *(Boron, pp 899–901, 906–907. Guyton, pp 732–733.)* Patients often experience a sense of fullness (early satiety), abdominal bloating, and nausea following a vagotomy of the antrum. The stomach has three important motor functions: storage, trituration, and emptying. The ability of the stomach to serve as a reservoir is characteristic of the orad stomach (gastric fundus and corpus). Upon ingestion of a mixed meal (liquids and solids) a vago-vagal-mediated reflex, the accommodation reflex, limits the rise in intragastric pressure in response to an increase in intragastric volume. Sectioning of the vagus nerve or gastric resection of the orad stomach abolishes the reflex and leads to an increased intragastric pressure with a resultant increase in the gastric emptying of liquids. Trituration, the mechanical breakdown of large, solid food particles into smaller particles, is essential for the gastric emptying of solids. Trituration is the result of rhythmical contractions characteristic of the gastric antrum. Normally, solids do not empty until they are smaller than 1 to 2 mm in diameter. Distension of the antrum initiates both local, enteric neural reflexes and long, vago-vagal reflexes that increase the strength of antral contractions and promote the gastric emptying of solids. The loss of vagal input to the antrum markedly impairs the emptying of solids and often leads to an early sense of fullness.

197. The answer is a. (*Boron, p 886.*) Electrical slow wave activity in the gastrointestinal tract appears to originate from specialized pacemaker cells (interstitial cells of Cajal) located between the longitudinal and circular muscle layers and within the submucosal and myenteric plexuses. These pacemaker cells input directly onto the smooth muscle and receive input from enteric nerves. Rhythmic, phasic contractions are characteristic of the gastric antrum and the small and large intestines.

198. The answer is e. (*Boron, pp 894–903. Guyton, pp 742–746.*) Maximal acid output may be increased in patients with duodenal ulcer disease. Gastric juice contains a number of secretions including HCl, intrinsic factor, pepsinogen, water, and electrolytes. Gastric secretion can be studied during the interdigestive (basal phase) or the digestive (cephalic, gastric, and intestinal phases of acid secretion) periods. Increased acid output is the result of neural (ACh), hormonal (gastrin), and paracrine (histamine) stimuli acting on the oxyntic cell. Feedback regulation (inhibition) of acid secretion occurs as the result of hydrogen ion–stimulated release of somatostatin from paracrine cells located near gastrin-containing antral G cells and as the result of the presence of chyme in the small intestine. The latter limits the secretion of acid via neural (enterogastric reflex) and hormonal (enterogastrone) pathways. Removal of intestinal inhibitory feedback leads to increased acid output. Enterooxyntin is a putative small intestinal hormone that stimulates gastric acid secretion.

199. The answer is a. *(Boron, pp 903–906. Guyton, pp 746–748.)* Pancreatic bicarbonate secretion into the small intestine is essential for neutralization of gastric acid emptied into the small intestine. Unlike the gastric mucosal lining, the mucosal surface of the small intestine does not evidence a significant endogenous defense mechanism against the insult of HCl. Upon delivery into the proximal small intestine, hydrogen ions stimulate the release of the hormone secretin from the intestinal wall, which in turn stimulates pancreatic bicarbonate secretion. In fact, the acid output of the stomach during a meal is matched equally by the pancreatic output of bicarbonate. Although the liver secretes bicarbonate and bile contains bicarbonate, the amounts are not sufficient for acid neutralization.

200. The answer is c. *(Boron, p 937. Guyton, pp 759–761.)* Absorption of bicarbonate from the small intestine occurs primarily in the jejunum and is the result of bicarbonate-stimulated Na/H exchange. In the presence of luminal bicarbonate, the activity of the exchanger increases and the resultant secreted hydrogen ion combines with bicarbonate to form carbon dioxide and water, which are subsequently absorbed. In addition to the exogenous dietary intake of bicarbonate, the ion is produced endogenously in salivary, gastric, intestinal, and hepatobiliary secretions.

201. The answer is d. *(Boron, pp 983–995.)* Bile acid synthesis is catalyzed by the microsomal enzyme 7α-hydroxylase. Bile is a complex mixture of inorganic and organic substances. The predominant organic component of bile is the bile salts, which make up about 67% of the total solutes. Primary bile acids, cholic acid and chenodeoxycholic acid, are synthesized from cholesterol. The rate-limiting step is catalyzed by the microsomal enzyme 7α-hydroxylase. Secondary bile acids, deoxycholic acid and lithocholic acid, are produced by biotransformation of primary bile acids by intestinal bacteria. Prior to secretion, the bile acids are conjugated with either glycine or taurine, which greatly enhances their water solubility.

202. The answer is b. *(Boron, pp 895–897. Guyton, pp 749–751.)* Withdrawal from long-term use of proton pump inhibitors prescribed for peptic ulcer disease may be associated with rebound gastric hypersecretion. Pharmacological suppression of gastric acid secretion can occur when the administered drug binds to a receptor present on the parietal cell or when it antagonizes the hydrogen-potassium-ATPase pump responsible for the active secretion of hydrogen ion into the gastric lumen. At the present time, the most effective antisecretory compounds work by blocking the histamine type-2 (H_2) receptor present on the parietal cell or by inhibition of the hydrogen pumps. The latter are the most potent and long-acting, thus increasing the probability of increasing serum gastrin.

203. The answer is b. *(Boron, pp 888–890.)* An intact enteric nervous system is essential for propagation of migrating motor complexes along the bowel. During the interdigestive period, the GI tract undergoes regular increases in peristaltic contractile activity about every 90 min that are termed migrating motor complexes. Originally recorded from the small intestine, they may begin in the smooth muscle of the esophagus or the stomach. They are commonly associated with periodic increases in the hormone motilin. Although it is still unclear, they appear to serve a "housekeeping function" by clearing the GI tract of luminal contents. They are immediately interrupted when a meal is ingested.

204. The answer is e. *(Boron, pp 888–889, 901, 921–923. Guyton, pp 733–734.)* The delivery of food into the proximal small intestine is accompanied by the appearance of segmenting intestinal contractions. The presence of food in the small intestine initiates neural reflexes and the release of hormones that affect a variety of gastrointestinal processes. The presence of food in the proximal small intestine is inhibitory to gastric secretion and emptying (enterogastric reflex, enterogastrone), stimulates pancreatic and hepatobiliary secretions (CCK, secretin), and increases small intestine segmentation. The latter is responsible for mixing chyme with bile and the digestive enzymes.

205. The answer is e. *(Boron, pp 1001, 1226.)* Vitamin K is a fat-soluble vitamin produced by intestinal bacteria that is essential for maintaining normal clotting of blood. The vitamin is essential for hepatic synthesis of prothrombin and factors VII, IX and X. Common causes of vitamin K deficiency include cholestasis, and factors that limit fat absorption.

206. The answer is b. (*Boron, pp 906–907.*) The orad (proximal) region of the stomach is responsible for the regulation of the liquid component of a meal. Delivery of food into the orad stomach activates an inhibitory vago-vagal reflex that promotes the reservoir function of the stomach (accommodation reflex). Resection of the orad stomach lessens the vagal input to the orad stomach and leads to an enhanced increase in intragastric pressure in response to an increase in intragastric volume. Intragastric pressure is the primary determinant of the rate of liquid emptying from the stomach.

207. The answer is a. (*Boron, pp 949–953.*) Lactase is a brush border enzyme that hydrolyzes milk sugar (lactose) into glucose and galactose. Patients with a lactase deficiency may experience diarrhea, cramps, and intestinal gas. The diarrhea and cramping reflect the osmotic effect of the sugar on water flux across the intestine. Colonic bacteria metabolize lactose to fatty acids, CO_2, and H_2.

208. The answer is c. (*Boron, pp 886–888.*) Reflux of gastric contents into the smooth-muscle region of the esophagus leads to the development of secondary esophageal peristasis, characterized by enteric nerve–initiated peristalsis, beginning at the site of irritation and LES relaxation. Primary peristalsis is initiated by the medullary swallowing center and is preceded by an oral-pharyngeal phase.

209. The answer is b. (*Boron, pp 992–993.*) The delivery of food into the small intestine is characterized by prompt emptying of the gallbladder, resulting from fat-induced release of cholecystokinin. Secretin stimulates pancreatic bicarbonate secretion. Enterogastrone is inhibitory to gastric function; glucagon is involved in nutrient metabolism; motilin is an inter-digestive hormone responsible for migrating motor complex activity.

210. The answer is d. (*Boron, pp 933–940.*) Osmotic equilibration of gastric contents emptied into the small intestine occurs in the duodenum. Water and electrolyte absorption occurs in both the small intestine and colon. Unlike the small intestine, however, the colon has a relatively limited daily absorptive capacity (approximately 6 L/day). The limited capacity is the result of the highly impermeable nature of the tight junctions connecting the colonic epithelial cells. Most water and electrolytes derive from endogenous gastrointestinal secretions and may reach 6 to 8 L/day. Regional differences occur along the small bowel and between the small bowel and colon with respect to the individual transport processes. For example, although there is net absorption of nutrients and water and electrolytes in the duodenum, the leaky nature of the tight junctions leads to rapid osmotic equilibration of chyme emptied from the stomach. Also, although potassium absorption occurs in the small intestine, net secretion may occur in the colon. Cholera toxin affects electroneutral sodium transport in the small intestine.

211. The answer is c. *(Boron, pp 894–901. Guyton, pp 628–640.)* Somatostatin is the principal paracrine secretion inhibitory to gastric acid secretion. As the free hydrogen ion concentration of the gastric lumen increases, the stimulus for continued acid secretion decreases. This negative feedback is mediated via somatostatin. Hydrogen ions release the somatostatin from antral SS cells, which in turn decreases gastrin release. Gastrin is the principal hormone released during a meal that is excitatory to gastric acid secretion. Somatostatin may also directly inhibit hydrogen ion secretion by the oxyntic cell.

212. The answer is e. *(Guyton, pp 742–744, 768–769.)* Analysis of serum electrolytes reveals low potassium (hypokalemia), low chloride (hypochloremia), and metabolic alkalosis. These abnormalities arise from two sources. First, gastric juice contains potassium and chloride in concentrations higher than found in the plasma. Loss of gastric juice through vomiting or drainage leads to depletion of these electrolytes from the plasma. Second, the metabolic abnormalities are exacerbated by the student's dehydration. Contraction of the vascular volume leads to orthostatic hypotension and the activation of renal mechanisms important for conserving volume. As a result, water, sodium, and bicarbonate are reabsorbed at the expense of increased potassium and hydrogen excretion.

213. The answer is b. *(Boron, pp 1078–1081. Guyton, pp 884–891.)* Insulin, a pancreatic hormone, decreases tissue lipolysis. The main function of insulin is to stimulate anabolic reactions involving carbohydrates, fats, proteins, and nucleic acids. Therefore, insulin increases glucose utilization while also stimulating lipogenesis and proteogenesis. By promoting glucose utilization by cells, insulin decreases the need for gluconeogenesis and ketogenesis.

214. The answer is d. *(Boron, pp 983–995.)* Although only small amounts of bile acids are lost in the stool each day, the loss represents the only route of elimination of cholesterol from the body. The predominant organic component of bile is the bile salts, which make up about 67% of the total solutes. Bile salts are amphiphilic molecules, that is, they exhibit both water and lipid solubility. Primary bile acids, cholic acid and chenodeoxycholic acid, are synthesized from cholesterol. Secondary bile acids, deoxycholic acid and lithocholic acid, are produced by biotransformation of primary bile acids by intestinal bacteria. Prior to secretion, the bile acids are conjugated with either glycine or taurine, which greatly enhances their water solubility. In general, taurine conjugates are more water-soluble than glycine conjugates.

215. The answer is a. *(Boron, p 945.)* The two major types of diarrhea are osmotic and secretory. Osmotic diarrhea is the result of excess solute in the lumen of the small intestine (undigested nutrients) or colon (laxatives). The excess solute produces a bulk flow of water into the lumen in volumes that eventually overwhelm the absorptive capacity of the gut. In osmotic diarrhea, stool osmolarity is greater than normal. Secretory diarrhea is the result of crypt cell secretion of an isosmotic chloride solution combined with inhibition of electroneutral NaCl absorption from the small intestine. Diarrhea is defined as the excretion of 200 grams or more of water in the stool per day.

216. The answer is c. *(Boron, pp 952–953.)* The transport protein responsible for the sodium-dependent glucose transport in the small intestine is termed the SGLT1. The absorption of glucose occurs through the coordinated action of transport proteins located in the brush border and basolateral membranes of the enterocyte. Glucose uptake into the enterocyte occurs primarily via the sodium-dependent SGLT1 secondary active transport mechanism. Exit from the enterocyte occurs by facilitated diffusion and is mediated by the membrane transporter, Glut-2. Glut-5 is the membrane transporter located on the apical portion of the enterocyte responsible for the facilitated entry of fructose into the cell.

217. The answer is e. (*Boron, pp 964–967. Guyton, pp 762–763.*) The colon is the major site for the generation and absorption of short-chain fatty acids. They are products of bacterial metabolism of undigested complex carbohydrates derived from fruits and vegetables. In addition to exhibiting trophic effects on the colonic mucosa, they are believed to promote sodium absorption from the colon. The mechanism of action remains controversial.

218. The answer is a. (*Boron, pp 964–967.*) Medium-chain triglycerides are hydrolyzed by lipases more rapidly than long-chain fatty acids and are much more water-soluble than long-chain triglycerides. Medium-chain triglycerides (MCTs) are fatty acids of 6 to 12 carbon chain lengths that are present in small amounts in the normal diet. MCTs are not utilized for resynthesis of triglycerides and therefore are not packaged into chylomicrons. Instead, they are released directly into the portal blood. Because they are readily absorbed, MCTs can be used in patients with a wide variety of GI diseases resulting in malabsorption.

Respiratory Physiology

Questions

DIRECTIONS: Each question below contains five suggested responses. Select the **one best** response to each question.

219. The basic respiratory rhythm is generated in the

a. Apneustic center
b. Nucleus parabrachialis
c. Dorsal medulla
d. Pneumotaxic center
e. Cerebrum

220. At the end of a quiet inspiration, alveolar pressure is normally

a. 240 cmH_2O
b. 24 cmH_2O
c. 0 cm H_2O
d. 14 cmH_2O
e. 140 cmH_2O

Questions 221–223

An 18-year-old girl with a nine-year history of wheezing on exertion is referred for pulmonary function tests. The diagram below represents the spirometry tracing of a forced vital capacity. Her total lung capacity was 110% of predicted.

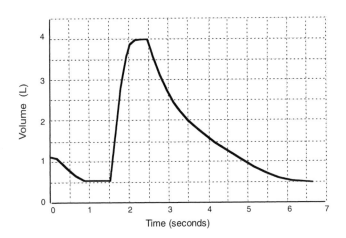

221. What is her FEV_1?

a. 1.5 L
b. 2.0 L
c. 2.5 L
d. 3.0 L
e. 3.5 L

222. The ratio of her FEV_1/FVC is approximately

a. 0.4 L
b. 0.5 L
c. 0.6 L
d. 0.7 L
e. 0.8 L

223. Which of the following values will most likely be above normal?

a. Vital capacity
b. Residual volume
c. Expiratory reserve volume
d. Maximum voluntary ventilation
e. Inspiratory capacity

Questions 224–227

A 40-year-old woman with a history of sinusitis and asthma since childhood presents to the emergency room with status asthmaticus and hypercapnic respiratory failure. She requires immediate intubation and mechanical ventilation and is treated with nebulized albuterol and IV methylprednisolone every 6 h. After muscle relaxation, on a control rate of 15 breaths/min and a tidal volume of 500 mL, the following values are obtained: $P_{A}CO_2 = 44$ mmHg, $F_{E}CO_2 = 2.8\%$.

224. Her Fa_{CO_2} is approximately

a. 0.40
b. 0.45
c. 0.50
d. 0.55
e. 0.60

225. Her physiological dead space is approximately

a. 140 mL
b. 180 mL
c. 220 mL
d. 260 mL
e. 300 mL

226. Her alveolar ventilation is approximately

a. 3000 mL/min
b. 3500 mL/min
c. 4000 mL/min
d. 4500 mL/min
e. 5000 mL/min

227. Her carbon dioxide production is approximately

a. 200 mL/min
b. 210 mL/min
c. 220 mL/min
d. 230 mL/min
e. 240 mL/min

Questions 228–229

A 26-year-old man presents to the emergency department with severe tonsillitis and a temperature of 103°F. The patient is in severe respiratory distress. Moderate amounts of pulmonary edema fluid are aspirated during suctioning. The patient is placed on a ventilator with an F_IO_2 of 0.5 and an arterial blood gas sample reveals a PO_2 of 160 mmHg and a PCO_2 of 40 mmHg.

228. His alveolar oxygen tension is approximately

a. 100 mmHg
b. 200 mmHg
c. 300 mmHg
d. 400 mmHg
e. 500 mmHg

229. Because recent clinical studies show that lower lung volumes during mechanical ventilation produce less lung damage, an attempt is made to reduce the tidal volume from 580 mL (11.1 mL/kg) to 450 mL (7.4 mL/kg) while keeping $PaCO_2$ at 40 mmHg. Assuming the patient has a physiological dead space of 180 mL, the respiratory rate should be changed from 16 breaths per minute to which of the following?

a. Approximately 20 breaths/min
b. Approximately 24 breaths/min
c. Approximately 28 breaths/min
d. Approximately 32 breaths/min
e. Approximately 36 breaths/min

Questions 230–231

A 68-year-old man who has COPD presents to his pulmonologist with fatigue, dyspnea at rest, and peripheral edema. His blood gases are Pa_{CO_2} = 30 mmHg, Pa_{O_2} = 60, and a pH of 7.6.

230. His alveolar-arterial (A - a) gradient is approximately

a. 10 mmHg
b. 20 mmHg
c. 30 mmHg
d. 40 mmHg
e. 50 mmHg

231. Which one of the following values is expected to be below normal in this patient?

a. Right atrial pressure
b. Hematocrit
c. Bicarbonate concentration
d. Alveolar ventilation
e. Diffusing capacity

Questions 232–233

The diagram below illustrates the intrapleural pressure generated by a patient who exhales forcefully.

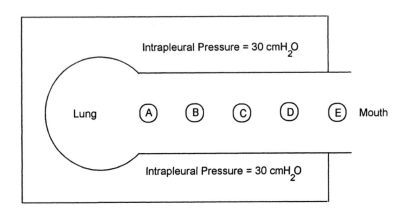

232. If the intrapleural pressure at the end of inspiration is 10 cmH$_2$O and the intrapleural pressure during expiration is 30 cmH$_2$O, the equal pressure point will be closest to point

a. A
b. B
c. C
d. D
e. E

233. The equal pressure point will move closer to the mouth if there is an increase in which of the following?

a. Airway resistance
b. Lung compliance
c. Lung volume
d. Expiratory effort
e. Airway smooth muscle tone

234. A healthy, 24-year-old man is prescribed sustained-release bupropion (Zyban) for smoking cessation. Twenty-one days after therapy he presents to his family physician with intermittent fever and a generalized rash, at which point the bupropion therapy is discontinued. A month later he develops a dry, intermittent cough and dyspnea. Blood gas analysis indicates a PaO_2 of 52 mmHg and a $PaCO_2$ of 32 mmHg. Which of the following pulmonary function test results is consistent with a diagnosis of allergic bronchospasm?

a. An increased forced vital capacity
b. A decreased FEV_1/FVC
c. An increased diffusing capacity
d. A decreased residual volume
e. An increased breathing frequency

235. A 27-year-old male presents to the emergency room with severe acute asthma. He reports that his symptoms began three days ago. Bronchodilator agents are administered and an arterial blood gas analysis reveals a non-anion gap metabolic acidosis. Which of the following conditions, all of which were present before he came to the emergency room, is responsible for the non-anion gap metabolic acidosis?

a. Dyspnea
b. Hypocapnia
c. Wheezing
d. Hypoxemia
e. Hyperinflation

236. A 5-month-old boy is admitted to the hospital for evaluation because of repeated episodes of sleep apnea. His ventilation did not increase when $PaCO_2$ was increased, but decreased during hyperoxia. Which of the following is the most likely cause of this infant's apnea?

a. Dysfunctional central chemoreceptors
b. Peripheral chemoreceptor hypersensitivity
c. Decreased irritant receptor sensitivity
d. Bronchial muscle spasm
e. Diaphragmatic fatigue

237. Which of the following values will decrease in a patient with ventilation-perfusion (V/Q) abnormalities?

a. Anion gap
b. Arterial pH
c. Arterial carbon dioxide tension
d. A - a gradient for oxygen
e. Alveolar ventilation

238. Which of the following is higher at the apex of the lung than at the base when a person is standing?

a. V/Q ratio
b. Blood flow
c. Ventilation
d. Pa_{CO_2}
e. Lung compliance

239. In areas of the lung with lower-than-normal V/Q ratios, the

a. Capillary CO_2 tension is lower than normal
b. Pulmonary vascular resistance is higher than normal
c. Alveolar O_2 tension is higher than normal
d. Water vapor pressure is higher than normal
e. Gas exchange ratio is higher than normal

240. Very small particles are removed from the respiratory system by which of the following?

a. Bulk flow
b. Diffusion
c. Expectoration
d. Phagocytosis
e. Ciliary transport

241. Which of the following conditions causes a decrease in arterial O_2 saturation without a decrease in O_2 tension?

a. Anemia
b. Carbon monoxide poisoning
c. A low V/Q ratio
d. Hypoventilation
e. Right-to-left shunt

242. The bulk of CO_2 is transported in arterial blood as which of the following?

a. Dissolved CO_2
b. Carbonic acid
c. Carbaminohemoglobin
d. Bicarbonate
e. Carboxyhemoglobin

243. A 27-year-old man presents to the emergency room with right heart failure and respiratory acidosis. Arterial blood gas analysis reveals a normal A - a gradient. Which of the following is the most likely cause of this patient's respiratory acidosis?

a. Left heart failure
b. Pulmonary edema
c. Airway obstruction
d. Hypoventilation
e. Anemia

244. At what point during the tidal breath illustrated below is the alveolar PCO_2 at its highest value?

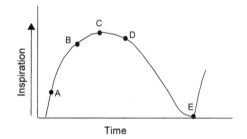

a. A
b. B
c. C
d. D
e. E

245. Peripheral and central chemoreceptors may both contribute to the increased ventilation that occurs as a result of which of the following?

a. A decrease in arterial oxygen content
b. A decrease in arterial blood pressure
c. An increase in arterial carbon dioxide tension
d. A decrease in arterial oxygen tension
e. An increase in arterial pH

246. Complete transection of the brainstem above the pons would

a. Result in cessation of all breathing movements
b. Prevent any voluntary holding of breath
c. Prevent the central chemoreceptors from exerting any control over ventilation
d. Prevent the peripheral chemoreceptors from exerting any control over ventilation
e. Abolish the Hering-Breuer reflex

Questions 247–248

The diagram below illustrates the change in intrapleural pressure during a single breath.

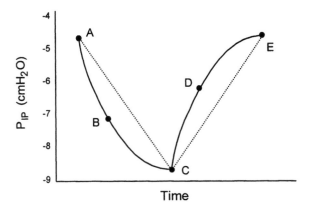

247. At which point on the diagram is inspiratory airflow the greatest?

a. A
b. B
c. C
d. D
e. E

248. At which point on the diagram is lung volume the greatest?

a. A
b. B
c. C
d. D
e. E

249. An 18-year-old girl presents to her primary care physician with an increased frequency of asthma exacerbations over the previous year. Her physical examination and the recording of her flow-volume loop (pictured below) are normal. At which point on the flow-volume loop will airflow remain constant despite an increased respiratory effort?

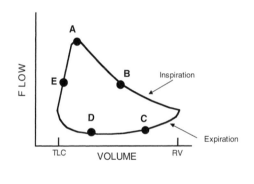

a. A
b. B
c. C
d. D
e. E

250. A 24-year-old woman develops adult respiratory distress syndrome (ARDS) after near-drowning due to attempted suicide. Conventional mechanical ventilation together with prone positioning and inhaled nitric oxide do not provide sufficient oxygenation. Porcine surfactant is instilled via fiberoptic bronchoscope, and the partial arterial carbon dioxide pressure ($PaCO_2$) and fraction of inspired oxygen (F_IO_2) ratio as well as shunt fraction (Qs/Qt) improve impressively. The improvements in respiratory function occurred because surfactant decreased which of the following?

a. Bronchiolar smooth-muscle tone
b. Arterial bicarbonate concentration
c. Lung compliance
d. The work of breathing
e. Functional residual capacity (FRC)

Questions 251–252

Use the following diagram to answer the questions.

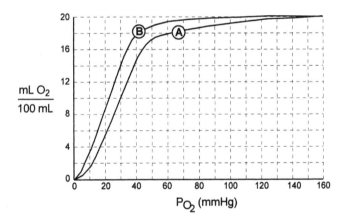

251. What is the P_{50} of the oxyhemoglobin curve labeled **A** in the diagram?

a. 80 mmHg
b. 60 mmHg
c. 40 mmHg
d. 30 mmHg
e. 20 mmHg

252. Which of the following conditions is most likely to shift the oxy-hemoglobin curve from **A** to **B**?

a. Increased temperature
b. Exercise
c. Acclimatization to high altitude
d. Hyperventilation
e. Metabolic acidosis

253. Which one of the following is higher at total lung capacity than it is at residual volume?

a. Anatomical dead space
b. Maximum static inspiratory pressure
c. Lung compliance
d. Airway resistance
e. Alveolar pressure

Questions 254–255

A 32-year-old male is hospitalized with severe respiratory disease following aspiration pneumonia. Inhaled nitric oxide is administered and he is placed in a prone position to improve oxygenation. Arterial and mixed venous blood gases are obtained after the administration of nitric oxide (data shown below).

254. Calculate the shunt fraction (the ratio of shunted to total pulmonary blood flow).

	After NO
Mean pulmonary capillary oxygen content	19 mL/dL
Arterial oxygen content	18 mL/dL
Mixed venous oxygen content	14 mL/dL

a. 10%
b. 20%
c. 30%
d. 40%
e. 50%

255. If the cardiac output of the patient in question 254 is 6 L/min, what is his oxygen consumption?

a. 200 mL/dL
b. 210 mL/dL
c. 220 mL/dL
d. 230 mL/dL
e. 240 mL/dL

256. A 37-year-old woman is admitted to the hospital with severe kyphoscoliosis (KS). KS is defined as a deformity of the spine involving both lateral displacement (scoliosis) and anteroposterior angulation (kyphosis). Over time, this anatomical distortion results in respiratory muscle weakness. Which of the following laboratory values will most likely be above normal in this patient?

a. Tidal volume
b. Oxyhemoglobin saturation
c. Vital capacity
d. Arterial carbon dioxide tension
e. Arterial pH

257. Measurement of the lecithin-sphingomyelin (L-S) ratio in amniotic fluid assesses which of the following?

a. The placenta's ability to oxygenate the fetus
b. Fetal adrenal function
c. Fetal kidney development
d. Fetal brain development
e. Fetal lung maturity

258. When the respiratory muscles are relaxed, the lungs are at

a. Residual volume (RV)
b. Expiratory reserve volume (ERV)
c. Functional residual capacity (FRC)
d. Inspiratory reserve volume (IRV)
e. Total lung capacity (TLC)

259. Which one of the following is the most likely cause of a high arterial P_{CO_2}?

a. Increased metabolic activity
b. Increased alveolar dead space
c. Depressed medullary respiratory centers
d. Alveolar capillary block
e. Increased alveolar ventilation

260. Pulmonary vascular resistance decreases if

a. The lungs are inflated to total lung capacity
b. Sympathetic stimulation to the pulmonary vessels is increased
c. Alveolar oxygen tension is decreased
d. Plasma hydrogen ion concentration is decreased
e. Cardiac output is increased

261. Which of the following would normally be less in the fetus than in the mother?

a. Pa_{CO_2}
b. Pulmonary vascular resistance
c. Affinity of hemoglobin for oxygen
d. Pa_{O_2}
e. Arterial hydrogen ion concentration

262. An increase in the P_{50} of an oxyhemoglobin curve would result from a decrease in which of the following?

a. Metabolism
b. pH
c. Temperature
d. Oxygen
e. 2,3-DPG

263. During moderate aerobic exercise,

a. Pa_{O_2} increases
b. Pa_{CO_2} decreases
c. Arterial pH decreases
d. Alveolar ventilation increases
e. Blood lactate level increases

264. A 29-year-old farmer develops a headache and becomes dizzy after working on a tractor in his barn. His wife suspects carbon monoxide poisoning and brings him to the emergency room where he complains of dizziness, lightheadedness, headache, and nausea. Arterial blood gas measurements reveal an elevated carboxyhemoglobin level. The patient does not appear to be in respiratory distress and denies dyspnea. The absence of respiratory signs and symptoms associated with carbon monoxide poisoning occurs because

a. Blood flow to the carotid body is decreased
b. Arterial oxygen content is normal
c. Cerebrospinal fluid pH is normal
d. Central chemoreceptors are depressed
e. Arterial oxygen tension is normal

265. Pulmonary alveoli are kept dry by factors that include the

a. Phagocytic activity of alveolar macrophages
b. Negative interstitial fluid pressure
c. Low vapor pressure of water in inspired air
d. Secretion of surfactant
e. Tight junctions between the alveolar capillary endothelial cells

266. In which one of the following conditions will the diffusing capacity of the lung increase?

a. Formation of pulmonary emboli
b. Fibrotic lung disease
c. Polycythemia
d. Congestive heart failure
e. COPD

267. The percentage of hemoglobin saturated with oxygen will increase if

a. The arterial P_{CO_2} is increased
b. The hemoglobin concentration is increased
c. The temperature is increased
d. The arterial P_{O_2} is increased
e. The arterial pH is decreased

268. Which of the following will return toward normal during acclimatization to high altitude?

a. Arterial hydrogen ion concentration
b. Arterial carbon dioxide tension
c. Arterial bicarbonate ion concentration
d. Arterial hemoglobin concentration
e. Alveolar ventilation

269. Which one of the following statements characterizes pulmonary compliance?

a. It decreases with advancing age
b. It is inversely related to the elastic recoil properties of the lung
c. It increases in patients with pulmonary edema
d. It is equivalent to DP/DV
e. It increases when there is a deficiency of surfactant

270. The activity of the central chemoreceptors is stimulated by which of the following?

a. An increase in the P_{CO_2} of blood flowing through the brain
b. A decrease in the P_{O_2} of blood flowing through the brain
c. A decrease in the oxygen content of blood flowing through the brain
d. A decrease in the metabolic rate of the surrounding brain tissue
e. An increase in the pH of the CSF

271. In an acclimatized person at high altitudes, oxygen delivery to the tissues may be adequate at rest because of

a. An increase in hemoglobin concentration
b. The presence of an acidosis
c. A decrease in the number of tissue capillaries
d. The presence of a normal arterial P_{O_2}
e. The presence of a lower-than-normal arterial P_{CO_2}

272. Which of the following will increase as a result of stimulating parasympathetic nerves to the bronchial smooth muscle?

a. Lung compliance
b. Airway diameter
c. Elastic work of breathing
d. Resistive work of breathing
e. Anatomic dead space

273. During a normal inspiration, more air goes to the alveoli at the base of the lung than to the alveoli at the apex of the lung because

a. The alveoli at the base of the lung have more surfactant
b. The alveoli at the base of the lung are more compliant
c. The alveoli at the base of the lung have higher V/Q ratios
d. There is a more negative intrapleural pressure at the base of the lung
e. There is more blood flow to the base of the lung

274. A spirometer can be used to measure directly

a. Functional residual capacity
b. Inspiratory capacity
c. Residual volume
d. Total lung capacity
e. Physiological dead space

275. Which of the following conditions is most likely to produce the change from the normal maximum flow-volume curve illustrated below?

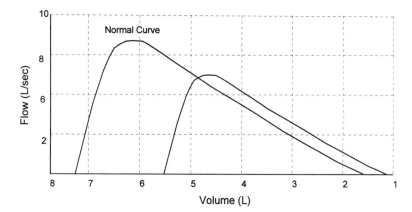

a. Asthma
b. Emphysema
c. Bronchiolitis
d. Fibrosis
e. Fatigue

276. The affinity of hemoglobin for oxygen is increased by which of the following?

a. Metabolic acidosis
b. Exercise
c. Hypoxemia
d. Anemia
e. Carbon monoxide poisoning

277. The oxygen consumption of the respiratory muscles is decreased by which of the following?

a. A decrease in lung compliance
b. A decrease in airway resistance
c. An increase in the rate of respiration
d. A decrease in the production of pulmonary surfactant
e. An increase in tidal volume

278. Which of the following characteristics is the most similar between the pulmonary and skeletal muscle capillaries?

a. The interstitial protein concentration
b. The interstitial hydrostatic pressure
c. The capillary oncotic pressure
d. The capillary hydrostatic pressure
e. The capillary permeability to proteins

279. An increase in pulmonary blood flow during exercise

a. Causes alveolar oxygen tension to decrease
b. Causes the V/Q ratio at the top of the lung to increase
c. Causes pulmonary arterial resistance to decrease
d. Causes diffusion capacity to decrease
e. Causes arterial oxygen saturation to decrease

280. Which one of the following will be greater than normal in a patient with a low V/Q ratio?

a. Pa_{CO_2}
b. Pa_{O_2}
c. A - a gradient
d. Oxygen dissolved in blood
e. Oxygen combined with hemoglobin

281. Which one of the following contributes to the normal difference between the alveolar and arterial oxygen tension (A - a) gradient?

a. The low P_{O_2} in the mixed venous blood
b. The inability of pulmonary capillary blood to equilibrate with alveolar gas
c. The low solubility of oxygen in blood
d. The shape of the oxyhemoglobin saturation curve
e. The high affinity of hemoglobin for oxygen in arterial blood

282. A patient with inadequate surfactant will have a relatively normal

a. FEV_1
b. FVC
c. FEV_1/FVC
d. MVV
e. V/Q ratio

283. Enzymes within the lung are responsible for the activation of which of the following?

a. Angiotensin II
b. Bradykinin
c. Prostaglandins
d. Serotonin
e. Leukotrienes

284. When a person ascends to a high altitude, alveolar ventilation increases. Alveolar ventilation continues to increase over the next several days because

a. The central chemoreceptors become more sensitive to low oxygen tensions
b. The peripheral chemoreceptors increase their firing rate
c. The plasma concentration of 2,3-DPG increases
d. The pH of the cerebrospinal fluid decreases
e. The oxygen-carrying capacity of hemoglobin increases

285. The clinical sign of cyanosis is caused by which of the following?

a. An increase in the affinity of hemoglobin for oxygen
b. A decrease in the percent of red blood cells (hematocrit)
c. An increase in the concentration of carbon monoxide in the venous blood
d. A decrease in the concentration of iron in the red blood cells
e. An increase in the concentration of deoxygenated hemoglobin

286. Which one of the following gases diffuses across the alveoli-capillary membrane by a diffusion-limited transport process?

a. Oxygen
b. Nitrogen
c. Carbon dioxide
d. Carbon monoxide
e. Nitrous oxide (N_2O)

287. Hyperventilation normally occurs during

a. Pregnancy
b. Sleep
c. Morphine administration
d. Exercise
e. Metabolic alkalosis

288. A person ascends to the top of a mountain where the atmospheric pressure is below normal. Which one of the following blood gases was most likely drawn from a person at the top of a mountain?

	P_{O_2}	P_{CO_2}
a.	50 mmHg	30 mmHg
b.	60 mmHg	40 mmHg
c.	80 mmHg	50 mmHg
d.	100 mmHg	40 mmHg
e.	120 mmHg	30 mmHg

289. Hyperventilation in response to a stressful situation leads to which of the following?

a. A decrease in the blood flow to the brain
b. An increase in the activity of the central chemoreceptors
c. A decrease in pH of the arterial blood
d. An increase in the resistance of the pulmonary blood vessels
e. A decrease in the excitability of nerve and muscle cells

290. Patients with chronic lung disease are often divided into "blue bloaters" (those who are cyanotic) and "pink puffers" (those who are not cyanotic). The presence of cyanosis in blue bloaters but not in pink puffers results from the difference in their

a. V/Q ratios
b. Vital capacities
c. Airway resistances
d. Total lung capacities
e. Expiratory flow rates

Questions 291–292

Use the following diagram of oxyhemoglobin saturation curves to answer the next two questions.

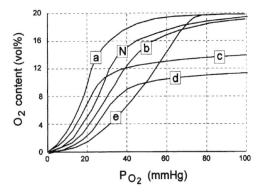

291. Which of the above oxyhemoglobin saturation curves was obtained from fetal blood?

a. A
b. B
c. C
d. D
e. E

292. Which of the oxyhemoglobin saturation curves was obtained from blood exposed to carbon monoxide?

a. A
b. B
c. C
d. D
e. E

Questions 293–294

A 72-year-old woman presents to her physician with dyspnea. The following data are obtained from the physical examination and arterial blood laboratory tests.

Heart rate   120 beats/min
Blood pressure   145/95 mmHg
H^+ 25 nM
Pa_{O_2} 60 mmHg
    Respiratory Rales Present

293. Which of the following values is most likely to be below normal?

a. Left atrial pressure
b. Pulmonary artery resistance
c. Pulmonary artery pressure
d. A – a gradient
e. Pa_{CO_2}

294. Providing oxygen to this patient increases her Pa_{O_2} to 90 mmHg. Which of the following values will most likely decrease?

a. H^+ ion concentration
b. Pulmonary artery resistance
c. Alveolar oxygen tension
d. Arterial carbon dioxide tension
e. A – a gradient

Questions 295–296

The following table shows several combinations of arterial blood-gas changes.

	pH	Paco$_2$	Pao$_2$
A.	↑	↑	↑
B.	↓	↑	↑
C.	↑	↑	↓
D.	↓	↓	↑
E.	↑	↓	↓

295. Which of the above changes in arterial blood gas values was obtained from a patient with a large intrapulmonary shunt?

a. A
b. B
c. C
d. D
e. E

296. Which of the above changes in arterial blood gas values was obtained from a patient with metabolic acidosis?

a. A
b. B
c. C
d. D
e. E

297. A 29-year-old male is admitted to the intensive care unit with pneumonia and requires supplemental oxygen. Lung function tests reveal: total lung capacity = 3.34 L (56% of predicted), residual volume = 0.88 L (54% of predicted), and force vital capacity = 1.38 L (30% of predicted). Which of the following characteristics will be approximately normal?

a. Lung compliance
b. Tidal volume
c. V/Q ratio
d. Diffusing capacity
e. FEV$_1$/FVC ratio

298. Airway resistance is lowest

a. During a forced expiration
b. At the total lung capacity
c. At the residual volume
d. During vagal stimulation
e. When breathing gas with low oxygen

Respiratory Physiology

Answers

219. The answer is c. *(Boron, pp 714–719. Guyton, pp 474–476.)* The basic respiratory rhythm originates from spontaneous rhythmic discharge of inspiratory neurons located in the respiratory center in the dorsal medulla. This basic rhythm can be modified by many factors, including voluntary control of breathing. In the pons are the apneustic center and the pneumotaxic center (which is located in the nucleus parabrachialis). These modify and regularize the basic respiratory rhythm to produce adequate breathing.

220. The answer is c. *(Boron, pp 626–629. Guyton, pp 432–434.)* During inspiration, the pressure in the alveoli (the alveolar pressure) becomes negative and gas is drawn into the lung by the difference in pressure between the alveoli and the atmosphere. At the peak of a normal inspiration, this pressure difference is only a few centimeters of water. At the end of inspiration, the pressure in the alveoli becomes equal to the atmospheric pressure, and flow ceases. During expiration, the alveolar pressure rises above atmospheric pressure and gas is expelled from the lungs. The alveolar pressure again equals atmospheric pressure at the end of expiration.

221–223. The answers are 221-b, 222-c, 223-b. *(Boron, pp 606–611. Guyton, pp 436–438.)* During a forced vital capacity (FVC), the patient is asked to breathe in as much air as possible and then expel all of the gas in her lung as fast as possible. The FEV_1 is the volume of gas expelled from the lung during the first second. The ratio of the FEV_1 to the FVC is, in this case, 2 L/3.5 L, which equals 0.57 (approximately 0.6). Obstructive diseases are characterized by a greater-than-normal total lung capacity (TLC), residual volume (RV), and functional residual capacity (FRC). The inspiratory and expiratory reserves (inspiratory capacity and expiratory volume) are decreased, as is the maximum voluntary ventilation.

224–227. The answers are 224-e, 225-d, 226-b, 227-c. *(Boron, pp 686–693.)* The FA_{CO_2} (the fraction of CO_2 in the alveolar gas) equals the ratio of partial pressure of CO_2 to the total dry atmospheric pressure $(P_{atm} - P_{water\ vapor} = (760 - 47)$ mmHg at sea level and body temperature.

$$F_{A}CO_2 = P_{A}CO_2/(P_{atm} - P_{water\ vapor}) = 44\ mmHg/(760 - 47)\ mmHg$$

$$F_{A}CO_2 = 44\ mmHg/(760 - 47)\ mmHg$$

$$F_{A}CO_2 = 0.06$$

The physiological dead space is calculated using Bohr's equation.

$$Dead\ Space = V_T \times \left(\frac{F_{A}CO_2 - F_{E}CO_2}{F_{A}CO_2} \right)$$

$$Dead\ Space = 500\ mL \times \left(\frac{0.6 - 0.28}{0.6} \right) = 267\ mL$$

Alveolar ventilation equals the tidal volume (V_T) minus the dead space volume (V_D) times the breathing frequency.

$$\dot{V}_A = (V_T - V_D) \times f$$

$$\dot{V}_A = (500\ mL - 267\ mL) \times 15\ breaths/min$$

$$\dot{V}_A = 3495\ mL/min$$

All of the carbon dioxide in the alveolar gas is derived from metabolism. Therefore, the carbon dioxide production equals the alveolar ventilation times the fraction of carbon dioxide in the alveolar gas.

$$\dot{V}CO_2 = (F_{A}CO_2) \times \dot{V}_A = 0.06 \times 3495\ mL/min = 210\ mL/min$$

228–229. The answers are 228-c, 229-b. *(Boron, pp 690–693.)* The alveolar oxygen tension is calculated using the modified alveolar gas equation: ($P_{A}O_2 = P_{I}O_2 - P_{A}CO_2/R$). The $P_{I}O_2$ (the partial pressure of the inspired gas) equals the fraction of oxygen in the dry atmospheric gas (0.5) times the dry atmospheric pressure (713 mmHg). R is the gas exchange ratio, which is nominally 0.8. However, when 100% oxygen is used, $R = 1.0$.

$$P_{A}O_2 = 0.5 \times (760 - 47)\ mmHg - \frac{40\ mmHg}{0.8}$$

$$P_{A}O_2 = 357\ mmHg - 50\ mmHg = 307\ mmHg$$

Paco$_2$ is inversely proportional to alveolar ventilation. Alveolar ventilation is, in turn, equal to the tidal volume: the dead space volume times the respiratory rate. Therefore

$$P_{A_{CO_2}} \times \dot{V}_A \text{ (Original)} = P_{A_{CO_2}} \times \dot{V}_A \text{ (Final)}$$

$$40 \text{ mmHg} \times (580 - 180) \text{ mL/min} \times 16 \text{ b/min}$$

$$= 40 \text{ mmHg} \times (450 - 180) \text{ mL/min} \times \text{frequency}$$

$$\text{Frequency} = \frac{40 \text{ mmHg} \times (580 - 180) \text{ mL/min} \times 16 \text{ b/min}}{40 \text{ mmHg} \times (450 - 180) \text{ mL/min}}$$

$$\text{Frequency} = 24 \text{ b/min}$$

230–231. The answers are 230-e, 231-e. (Boron, pp 669–673, 684, 710). The A − a gradient is the partial pressure difference between the alveolar and arterial oxygen tensions. The arterial blood gas tension has been measured. The alveolar oxygen tension must be calculated using the modified alveolar gas equation

$$P_{A_{O_2}} = 0.21 \times (760 - 47) \text{ mmHg} - \frac{30 \text{ mmHg}}{0.8}$$

$$P_{A_{O_2}} = 150 \text{ mmHg} - 37.5 \text{ mmHg} = 112.5 \text{ mmHg}$$

$$(A - a)_{oxygen} \text{ gradient} = 113 \text{ mmHg} - 60 \text{ mmHg} = 53 \text{ mmHg}$$

The patient's low arterial oxygen tension results from a decrease in diffusion capacity and V/Q abnormalities. The resulting hypoxemia will lead to an increase in red blood cell production and therefore an increase in hematocrit. The low oxygen will also cause an increase in pulmonary vascular resistance and therefore an increase in right atrial pressure. Hypoxemia will also lead to an increase in alveolar ventilation and a respiratory alkalosis, which will be compensated for by an increase in bicarbonate concentration.

232. The answer is b. (Boron, pp 629–632.) The equal pressure point is the point at which the pressure inside the airways equals the intrapleural pressure. If the equal pressure point occurs where the bronchioles can collapse, the airway will narrow and the maximum expiratory flow rate will be limited. The intra-airway pressure at the beginning of the airways (closest to the alveoli) equals the sum of the recoil pressure (exerted by the alveoli) and the intrapleural pressure (produced by the muscles of expiration). Therefore, the intra-airway pressure at the alveoli equals 40 cmH_2O (10 cm H_2O plus 30 cmH_2O). Assuming that the intra-airway pressure is zero at the mouth and drops linearly from the alveoli to the mouth, the intra-airway pressure will be 30 cmH_2O one-fourth of the way down the airway (point **B**), 20 cmH_2O one-half of the way down the airway, and 10 cmH_2O three-fourths of the way down the airway. Since the intrapleural pressure is 30 cmH_2O, the equal pressure point will be approximately one-fourth of the way down the airway (point **B**).

233. The answer is c. *(Boron, pp 629–632.)* The equal pressure point moves further away from the lungs if the recoil force is increased and moves closer to the lungs when the intrapleural pressure is increased. Increasing the lung volume expands the alveoli and makes their recoil force greater. This moves the equal pressure point toward the mouth. If airway resistance increases, for example, by increasing airway smooth muscle tone, then a greater expiratory effort and consequently a greater intrapleural pressure will be necessary to expel the gas from the lungs.

234. The answer is b. *(Boron, pp 606–608, 624–625.)* Bronchospasm increases the resistance to airflow, which makes it more difficult to expel gas rapidly from the lung during expiration, so although both FEV_1 and vital capacity decreases, the percent of gas expelled in 1 s as a function of the total amount that can be expelled (the FEV_1/FVC ratio) also decreases dramatically. Obstructive disease also produces air trapping, so all static lung volumes, residual volume, functional residual capacity, and total lung capacity will increase.

235. The answer is b. *(Boron, pp 640–646, 730.)* During the early stages of an asthmatic attack, patients often hyperventilate, producing a decrease in arterial CO_2 concentration (hypocapnia). Over 3 days, the kidneys compensate for the respiratory alkalosis by lowering bicarbonate. When the respiratory problem is resolved, the patient will be left with a metabolic acidosis and a normal anion gap. Hypoxemia may, in some cases, produce a lactic acidosis, which is accompanied by an increased anion gap.

236. The answer is a. *(Boron, pp 713–714, 723–731.)* The central chemoreceptors respond to changes in P_{CO_2} and, more slowly, to changes in pH. The failure of CO_2 to increase ventilation indicates that the central chemoreceptors are not functioning properly. The peripheral chemoreceptors respond to hypoxia, hypercapnia, and acidemia. Because ventilation decreased when P_{O_2} was increased (hyperoxia), the peripheral chemoreceptors are most likely the primary driving force for ventilation. Bronchial muscle spasm can produce airway obstruction and if severe enough prevent ventilation but is not likely to be a cause of periodic episodes of apnea. Although diaphragmatic fatigue can decrease ventilation, the accessory muscles of respiration will prevent apnea from occurring.

237. The answer is c. *(Boron, pp 702–711. Guyton, pp 460–461.)* V/Q mismatches will cause arterial oxygen levels (Pa_{O_2}) to decrease. Decreased Pa_{O_2} will stimulate the peripheral chemoreceptors, which, in turn, will increase alveolar ventilation and decrease Pa_{CO_2}. The decreased Pa_{CO_2} will cause a respiratory alkalosis (increasing pH). Hypoxemia will also cause lactate levels to rise, increasing the anion gap (and blunting the rise in pH). The fall in Pa_{O_2} causes the A − a gradient to rise.

238. The answer is a. *(Boron, pp 702–711. Guyton, pp 460–461.)* The alveoli at the apex of the lung are larger than those at the base so their compliance is less. Because the compliance is reduced, less inspired gas goes to the apex than to the base. Also, because the apex is above the heart, less blood flows through the apex than through the base. However, the reduction in airflow is less than the reduction in blood flow, so that the V̇/Q̇ ratio at the top of the lung is greater than it is at the bottom. The increased V̇/Q̇ ratio at the apex makes $P_{A_{CO_2}}$ lower and $P_{A_{O_2}}$ higher at the apex than they are at the base.

239. The answer is b. *(Boron, pp 702–711. Guyton, pp 460–461.)* Proper gas exchange requires an appropriate matching of ventilation and blood flow referred to as the V̇/Q̇ ratio. If perfusion (Q̇) exceeds ventilation (V̇), the amount of oxygen diffusing into the capillary blood and the amount of carbon dioxide diffusing out of the capillary blood is reduced. The result is a lower-than-normal P_{O_2} and a higher-than-normal CO_2. The lower P_{O_2} will cause vascular resistance to rise above normal.

240. The answer is d. *(Boron, pp 604–605. Guyton, pp 440–442.)* The lung has a variety of mechanisms to remove particulate matter from the inspired gas. Large particles become deposited in the mucus layer that lies within the bronchi. The mucus is swept up and out of the bronchioles by the ciliated epithelial cells that line the bronchioles. Smaller particles remain suspended in the inspired gas and reach the alveoli. Alveolar macrophages remove these particles by phagocytosis. The macrophages are usually removed from the lung through the lymphatic or blood circulation. Cigarette smoking can prevent cilia from beating, reduce macrophage migration, and thus impair the ability of the lungs to remove potentially harmful particles inhaled from the atmosphere.

241. The answer is b. *(Boron, pp 663, 673–674.)* A rise or fall in the oxygen saturation of hemoglobin is caused by a decrease in the arterial O_2 tension, which can result from a low V/Q ratio, hypoventilation, or an anatomical right-to-left shunt. Because carbon monoxide (CO) competes with O_2 on the hemoglobin molecule, CO poisoning can cause a decrease in hemoglobin's saturation even when the P_{O_2} is normal. In anemia, oxygen saturation is unchanged but the concentration of hemoglobin is less than normal, reducing the oxygen content.

242. The answer is d. *(Boron, pp 663–665. Guyton, pp 470–472.)* CO_2 is transported in arterial blood in three forms: as physically dissolved CO_2 (about 5%), in combination with the amino groups of hemoglobin as carbaminohemoglobin (about 5%), and as bicarbonate ion HCO_3^- (about 90%). The amount of CO_2 actually carried as carbonic acid, H_2CO_3, is negligible. Carboxyhemoglobin refers to the combination of carbon monoxide (CO) and hemoglobin.

243. The answer is d. *(Boron, pp 692, 730–731.)* Hypoventilation produces a rise in arterial P_{CO_2}, which causes a respiratory acidosis. Renal compensation for a respiratory acidosis results in an increase in bicarbonate and a decrease in chloride concentration, which results in a normal anion gap. Left heart failure is a common cause of right heart failure and of pulmonary edema but neither will produce a pure respiratory acidosis. If the pulmonary edema or reduction in cardiac output is severe enough, a metabolic acidosis could result from anaerobic metabolism.

244. The answer is a. (*Boron, pp 686–690.*) The alveolar P_{CO_2} rises and falls with each breath. As CO_2 diffuses into the alveoli from the blood, the alveolar P_{CO_2} rises. The P_{CO_2} falls when fresh air is added to the alveolar gas. The highest P_{CO_2} occurs just before fresh air is inhaled. The first gas entering the alveoli during inspiration is actually alveolar gas because the conducting airways are filled with alveolar gas at the end of expiration. Fresh air does not enter the alveoli until the alveolar gas has been emptied from the dead space. In normal tidal breathing, dead space volume is approximately 30% of tidal volume. Therefore, the alveolar P_{CO_2} continues to rise for the first one-third of each breath and reaches its highest value at the point labeled **A**.

245. The answer is c. (*Boron, pp 712–714, 723–731.*) The central chemoreceptors located on or near the ventral surface of the medulla cause an increase in ventilation in response to an increase in Pa_{CO_2} and to a lesser extent to a decrease in arterial pH because the blood-brain barrier is relatively impermeable to hydrogen ions. The peripheral chemoreceptors in the carotid bodies cause an increase in ventilation in response to an increase in Pa_{CO_2}, a decrease in arterial pH, and a decrease in Pa_{O_2}. Neither the central chemoreceptors nor the carotid bodies are stimulated by a decrease in arterial blood pressure or O_2 content.

246. The answer is b. (*Boron, pp 714–722. Guyton, pp 475–476.*) Transection of the brainstem above the pons would prevent any voluntary changes in ventilation by cutting the pathways from the higher centers. Breathing would continue because the pontine-medullary centers that control rhythmic ventilation would be intact. Inputs to the brainstem from the central and peripheral chemoreceptors that stimulate ventilation and from lung stretch receptors that inhibit inspiration (Hering-Breuer reflex) would also be intact and these reflexes would be maintained.

247–248. The answers are 247-b, 248-c. *(Boron, pp 606–608, 626–628.)* During inspiration (curve **ABC**), the respiratory muscles pull the chest wall out and diaphragm down and intrapleural pressure (P_{IP}) becomes more negative. The muscles must overcome the elastic recoil forces of the lungs and the resistance of the airways to airflow. The P_{IP} necessary to overcome the elastic forces of the lung is depicted by dashed line **AC**. The P_{IP} necessary to overcome the airway resistance is the difference between dashed line **AC** and curve **ABC**. The maximum airflow occurs at point **B**, where the difference between the two is the greatest. Lung volume is the greatest at point **C**, where P_{IP} is the most negative.

249. The answer is b. *(Boron, pp 629–632.)* The initial expiratory flow is effort-dependent. That is, increasing expiratory effort will increase expiratory flow. The remainder of the expiratory flow is effort-independent; once maximum flow rates are achieved, increasing effort will not produce an increased flow rate. The inability to increase flow rates is caused by airway compression. The pressure within the airways decreases from the lungs to the mouth. The pressure outside the airways, at any given lung volume, is the same throughout the thoracic cavity. Somewhere along the airways, an equal pressure point is reached at which the pressure inside and outside the airways is the same. If this point occurs at a region of the airways where compression can occur, it will limit the maximum flow. Increasing effort increases compression so that increased airway resistance counteracts the increased effort and no increase in flow occurs. This limitation of flow due to compression is referred to as the effort-independent portion of the flow-volume curve. It characterizes all but the initial portion of expiration. No effort limitation occurs during inspiration because increased expiratory efforts make the intrathoracic cavity more negative, which expands the airways, lowering their resistance.

250. The answer is d. *(Boron, pp 603, 616–621.)* Surfactant is composed of a lipid called dipalmitoylphosphatidylcholine and a variety of proteins. It reduces the surface tension (increases the compliance) of the lung and makes it easier for the lung to expand, thereby reducing the work of breathing. Without surfactant, the respiratory muscles may not be able to produce adequate ventilation, leading to hypercapnia and hypoxia. The increase in compliance results in an increase in FRC. The patient's acid-base status will improve and bicarbonate will return toward normal. Bronchiole smooth muscle tone may have contributed to the ventilatory difficulties of the patient but the inability of NO to improve her condition indicates that the primary problem was not related to airway constriction.

251–252. The answers are 251-d, 252-d. (*Boron, pp 656–663.*) The P_{50} of the oxyhemoglobin curve is the oxygen tension at which half of the hemoglobin is saturated with oxygen. When fully saturated, the hemoglobin represented by curve **A** has an oxygen content of 20 mL/dL. Therefore, the P_{50} is the P_{O_2} at which the hemoglobin contains one-half of 20 mL/dL (10 mL/dL), which is 30 mmHg. The oxyhemoglobin curve shifts to the left when pH is increased. Hyperventilation will decrease P_{CO_2} and cause an increase in pH. Increased temperature, decreased pH, and increased concentration of 2,3-DPG can shift the oxyhemoglobin dissociation curve to the right. Exercise will cause the temperature of the working muscles to increase and right-shift the oxyhemoglobin dissociation curve of the blood flowing through the working muscles. When a person remains at altitude for several days, the 2,3-DPG concentrations increase as part of the acclimatization process.

253. The answer is a. (*Boron, pp 687–690.*) Expanding the lungs lowers the intrathoracic pressure, which causes the airways to expand. Expanding the airways increases their volume and, therefore, the volume of the anatomical dead space. Expanding the airways also causes a decrease in airway resistance. Maximum static inspiratory pressure is maximal at function residual volume and decreases as lung volume is increased. Lung compliance is decreased; that is, the lungs are stiffer at high lung volumes. Alveolar pressure is atmospheric at residual volume and at total lung capacity.

254–255. The answers are 254-b, 255-e. (*Boron, pp 441–442, 671–673, 705–711.*) The fraction of the pulmonary blood flowing bypassing the lung (the shunt, Q_S) compared to the total pulmonary blood flow (Q_T) is calculated using the equation

$$\frac{Q_S}{Q_T} = \frac{C_cO_2 - C_aO_2}{C_cO_2 - C_{\bar{v}}O_2} = \frac{19 \text{ mL/dL} - 18 \text{ mL/dL}}{19 \text{ mL/dL} - 14 \text{ mL/dL}} = 0.2$$

$C_{c'}$ is the end pulmonary capillary blood oxygen content, C_aO_2 is the arterial oxygen content, and $C\bar{v}O_2$ is the mixed venous oxygen content. The oxygen consumption can be calculated if the cardiac output (CO) and the difference between the arterial and venous oxygen content are known using the equation

$$\dot{V}O_2 = CO \times (A - V)_{O_2 \text{ content}}$$

$$\dot{V}O_2 = 6 \text{ L/min} \times (18 \text{ mL/dL} - 14 \text{ mL/dL})$$

$$\dot{V}O_2 = 240 \text{ mL/min}$$

This method of calculating the oxygen consumption is called Fick's principle or Fick's method. It can also be used to calculate the cardiac output if the oxygen consumption and the difference between the arterial and venous oxygen content are known.

256. The answer is d. (*Boron, pp 641, 693–694, 729.*) Muscle weakness can produce inadequate ventilation, which can lead to an accumulation of carbon dioxide, a decrease in hemoglobin saturation, and a decrease in arterial pH. This type of respiratory disease is referred to as restrictive lung disease and is characterized by a decrease in tidal volume and vital capacity.

257. The answer is e. (*Boron, pp 603, 616–621.*) Lecithin (phosphatidylcholine) and sphingomyelin are choline phospholipids found in a variety of tissues. Lecithin is a major component of surfactant and its synthesis increases as the fetus matures and the lungs are prepared for expansion. Surfactant, a lipoprotein mixture, prevents alveolar collapse by permitting the surface tension of the alveolar lining to vary during inspiration and expiration. Thus, measurement of the lecithin-sphingomyelin (L-S) ratio in amniotic fluid provides an index of fetal lung maturity.

258. The answer is c. (*Boron, pp 606–608, 626–628. Guyton, pp 436–438.*) The lungs tend to recoil inward, whereas the chest wall tends to recoil outward. When the respiratory muscles are all relaxed, these two opposing forces are balanced. The volume of gas in the lungs at this point is the relaxation volume, or FRC.

259. The answer is c. *(Boron, pp 712–719, 725–726. Guyton, pp 476–479.)* A high arterial P_{CO_2} is most likely caused by depressed medullary respiratory centers. Depression of these centers decreases alveolar ventilation and results in hypoventilation with an increased Pa_{CO_2} and decreased Pa_{O_2}. This depression can be caused by drugs such as barbiturates or narcotics. Slight depression also occurs during sleep. If metabolic activity increases, as during mild exercise, alveolar ventilation increases in parallel and Pa_{CO_2} does not change. Retention of CO_2 could result from alveolar capillary block, but it would have to be extremely severe because CO_2 is so soluble in tissue.

260. The answer is e. *(Boron, pp 696–699.)* Pulmonary vascular resistance is affected by cardiac output, pulmonary artery pressure, lung volume, and O_2 tension. Increasing cardiac output or pulmonary artery pressure causes the pulmonary vasculature to expand, thereby decreasing PVR. At high lung volumes, intrapulmonary blood vessels are stretched and compressed, increasing PVR. At low lung volumes, extrapulmonary blood vessels are compressed, increasing PVR. The lowest PVR occurs near FRC. Decreasing P_{O_2} or increasing P_{CO_2} or H^+ concentration causes PVR to rise. The sympathetic nervous system has little direct effect on PVR.

261. The answer is d. *(Boron, pp 656–663, 1195–2000. Guyton, pp 946–947.)* Because fetal hemoglobin (hemoglobin F) is chemically different from adult hemoglobin in that it has two α and two γ chains instead of two α and two β chains, it has a greater affinity for oxygen. This is advantageous in the placental exchange of O_2 from maternal blood (Pa_{O_2} = 100 mmHg) to fetal blood (Pa_{O_2} = 25 mmHg). Pa_{CO_2} is about 2 to 3 mmHg higher in the fetus than in the mother. Arterial H^+ concentration is about the same in both. Pulmonary vascular resistance is high in the fetus, shunting blood away from the lungs. It decreases at birth and remains low.

262. The answer is b. *(Boron, pp 656–663.)* The P_{50} indicates the affinity of hemoglobin for O_2. A decrease in affinity results in an increase in the P_{50}. Hemoglobin's affinity for O_2 is decreased by a decrease in pH (an increase in H^+ concentration), an increase in temperature, and an increase in 2,3-DPG concentrations.

263. The answer is d. (*Boron, pp 1244–1252.*) During moderate aerobic exercise, oxygen consumption and CO_2 production increase, but alveolar ventilation increases in parallel. Thus, Pa_{O_2} and Pa_{CO_2} do not change. Arterial pH does not decrease and blood lactate concentration does not increase during moderate aerobic exercise, but arterial pH does decrease and blood lactate concentration does increase during anaerobic exercise because of increased production of lactic acid.

264. The answer is e. (*Boron, p 663.*) Carbon monoxide poisoning reduces the amount of oxygen that can combine with hemoglobin but does not reduce the arterial oxygen tension. Because the peripheral chemoreceptors do not increase ventilation until the arterial P_{O_2} is less than 60 mmHg, severe hypoxemia can occur without any respiratory or cardiovascular symptoms being apparent to the victim of CO poisoning. This is the reason that it is so important to install carbon monoxide detectors in homes and businesses.

265. The answer is b. (*Boron, pp 473, 600–601.*) The forces tending to remove fluid from the alveoli are the negative interstitial fluid pressure and the osmotic pressure exerted at the alveolar membrane by ions and crystalloid molecules in the interstitial fluid. Fluid movement into pulmonary capillaries, however, is a function of plasma oncotic pressure. The pulmonary capillaries are actually more permeable than those in the systemic circulation; that is, they have a higher hydraulic conductivity. Alveolar phagocytes do not take up significant amounts of water, and very little water from the alveoli goes into inspired air because the air is well humidified by the upper airways. Surfactant lowers the surface tension in the alveoli but does not affect fluid movement.

266. The answer is c. (*Boron, pp 674–682. Guyton, pp 458–460.*) In the tissues, the diffusing capacity is the volume of gas transported across the lung per minute per mmHg partial pressure difference. It is determined by the surface area and the thickness of the alveolar-capillary interface. Increases in the diffusing capacity can be produced by opening pulmonary capillaries, expanding the surface area of the pulmonary capillaries, optimizing the V/Q ratio within the lung, or by increasing the concentration of hemoglobin within the blood (polycythemia). It can be decreased by mismatching of ventilation and perfusion, pulmonary edema, or pulmonary emboli, all of which interfere with gas diffusion.

267. The answer is d. (Boron, pp 656–663. Guyton, pp 466–469.) The percentage of hemoglobin saturated with oxygen depends on the level of Po_2 in the blood and on other factors that affect the position of the oxyhemoglobin dissociation curve. Factors that shift the curve to the left, such as a decrease in Pco_2, an increase in pH, or a decrease in temperature, would increase the percentage of hemoglobin saturated with oxygen as would an increase in Po_2, provided that the percentage of saturation was not already at 100%. At a given Po_2, increasing the concentration of hemoglobin would not affect the percentage of saturation but would increase the oxygen content of the blood.

268. The answer is a. (Boron, pp 1262–1265. Guyton, pp 497–501.) At high altitude, the barometric pressure is reduced, resulting in a decrease in Pio_2, which decreases both alveolar and arterial Po_2. If Pao_2 is less than 60 mmHg, the carotid bodies are stimulated and cause hyperventilation, which increases alveolar ventilation and decreases $Paco_2$, with a resultant respiratory alkalosis. During acclimatization, Pao_2 remains low, ventilation remains high, and therefore $Paco_2$ remains low. The kidneys act to lower plasma bicarbonate and return arterial pH toward normal. The oxygen content of arterial blood increases, owing to an increase in hematocrit stimulated by the increased production of erythropoietin in the kidney.

269. The answer is b. (Boron, pp 611–618.) Pulmonary compliance, defined as the ratio of change of lung volume to the change in pressure required to inflate the lung ($\Delta V/\Delta P$), is an index of lung distensibility. It decreases in patients with pulmonary edema and interstitial fibrosis and increases in patients with emphysema and in persons of advancing years. The stiffer the lung is, the lower the pulmonary compliance. Surfactant lowers the surface tension in the alveoli and makes the lung more distensible.

270. The answer is a. (Boron, pp 712–714, 723–729. Guyton, pp 476–479.) The central chemoreceptors are located at or near the ventral surface of the medulla. They are stimulated to increase ventilation by a decrease in the pH of their extracellular fluid (ECF). The pH of this ECF is affected by the Pco_2 of the blood supply to the medullary chemoreceptor area as well as by the CO_2 and lactic acid production of the surrounding brain tissue. The central chemoreceptors are not stimulated by decreases in Pao_2 or blood oxygen content but rather can be depressed by long-term or severe decreases in oxygen supply.

271. The answer is a. *(Boron, pp 1262–1265. Guyton, pp 497–501.)* At a high altitude, arterial P_{O_2} is low because of the low barometric pressure. Ventilation increases owing to stimulation of the carotid body chemoreceptors, and Pa_{O_2} increases somewhat, although it does not return to a normal, sea-level value. Hyperventilation causes a decrease in Pa_{CO_2}, resulting in a respiratory alkalosis that may become fully compensated with time via renal mechanisms. A lower-than-normal Pa_{CO_2} would shift the oxyhemoglobin dissociation curve to the left, thereby increasing the affinity of hemoglobin for oxygen. Chronic hypoxia at high altitudes or in disease states stimulates the increased release of erythropoietin from the kidneys, which increases the hematocrit and thereby increases the hemoglobin concentration of the blood. Thus, at the same lowered Pa_{O_2}, the oxygen content of blood and oxygen delivery to tissues increase. Chronic hypoxia also stimulates increased capillary growth in tissues.

272. The answer is d. *(Boron, pp 621–625. Guyton, pp 440–441.)* The tone of bronchial smooth muscle is under autonomic control. Stimulation of sympathetic nerves causes bronchodilation, whereas parasympathetic stimulation via the vagus nerve causes bronchoconstriction. Bronchoconstriction reduces the radius of the airways and thereby decreases anatomic dead space and increases airway resistance, which consequently increases the resistive work of breathing. Bronchoconstriction has no significant effect on the elastic properties of the lung.

273. The answer is b. *(Boron, pp 700–704.)* There is a negative, or subatmospheric, intrapleural pressure (P_{IP}) between the lungs and the chest wall due to the tendency of the chest wall to pull outward and the tendency of the lungs to collapse. Because the lungs are essentially "hanging" in the chest, the force of gravity on the lungs causes the P_{IP} to be more negative at the top of the lung. This also causes the alveoli at the apex (top) of the lung to be larger than those at the base (bottom) of the lung. Larger alveoli are already more inflated and are less compliant than smaller alveoli. During inspiration, when all alveoli are subjected to essentially the same alveolar pressure, more air will go to the more compliant alveoli. Because of the effect of gravity on blood, more blood flow will go to the base of the lung. This does not appreciably affect lung compliance. Ventilation is about three times greater at the base of the lung, but flow is about 10 times greater at the base than at the apex of the lung. Therefore, the $\dot{V}/\dot{Q}$ ratio is lower at the base than at the apex in a normal lung.

274. The answer is b. (*Boron, pp 606–611.*) A spirometer is an instrument that records the volume of air moved into and out of the lungs during respiration and therefore can only be used to measure changes in lung volumes. It cannot be used to measure absolute lung volumes. The inspiratory capacity is the maximal amount of gas that can be inhaled when the lung volume is at its functional residual capacity (FRC). Therefore, changes in lung volume can be measured by spirometry, as can tidal volume, expiratory reserve volume, and vital capacity. The absolute lung volumes, residual volume, functional residual capacity, and total lung capacity cannot be measured directly by spirometry. Although the anatomical dead space can be estimated directly from spirometry if the subject breathes in a breath of pure oxygen, the physiological dead space, which is the combination of anatomical and alveolar dead spaces, can only be measured indirectly using a spirometer.

275. The answer is d. (*Boron, pp 629–632.*) The maximum flow-volume curve represents the greatest flow that can be produced at each volume during expiration. Muscular effort, lung recoil, and airway resistance affect the expiratory flow rate. Lung compliance decreases in fibrosis. The low lung compliance increases the recoil force at any given lung volume, and, therefore, the maximum flow rate at any given lung volume is higher than normal. Maximum flows are decreased in asthma and bronchiolitis because airway resistance has increased, in emphysema and bronchiolitis because lung recoil force has decreased, and in fatigue because muscular effort has decreased.

276. The answer is e. (*Boron, pp 659–663.*) Hemoglobin's O_2 affinity is increased by carbon monoxide. In carbon monoxide poisoning, carbon monoxide not only displaces O_2 from hemoglobin, it also makes it more difficult for the O_2 that is bound to hemoglobin (Hb) to dissociate from it in the tissues. Increasing H^+ ion concentration (decreasing pH) by metabolic acidosis or respiratory acidosis (decreased alveolar ventilation) decreases the affinity of hemoglobin for O_2. Exercise decreases the affinity of Hb for O_2 by increasing the temperature of the exercising muscles. Anemia has no direct effect on Hb affinity for oxygen, but if it results in tissue hypoxemia, it will cause an increase in 2,3-DPG, which decreases the affinity of Hb for O_2.

277. The answer is b. *(Boron, pp 621–631.)* Respiratory muscles consume oxygen in proportion to the work of breathing, which can be divided into resistance work and elastic work. Resistance work includes work to overcome tissue as well as airway resistance. A decrease in the amount of pulmonary surfactant would decrease lung compliance and increase the elastic work of breathing. An increase in respiratory rate increases the work of breathing.

278. The answer is c. *(Boron, pp 465–475, 695–696. Guyton, pp 166–170, 448–450.)* Blood flows in series through the systemic and pulmonary circulations, and, therefore, blood perfusing the skeletal muscles has the same oncotic pressure as the blood flowing through the pulmonary circulation. However, the blood pressure is much lower in the pulmonary circulation than in the systemic circulation, and because the thoracic cavity has a negative pressure, the interstitial fluid pressure is more negative in the pulmonary circulation than in the systemic circulation. The pulmonary capillaries are more permeable to proteins than the skeletal muscle capillaries, and, therefore, the interstitial concentration of protein is greater in the pulmonary circulation.

279. The answer is c. *(Boron, pp 697–698. Guyton, pp 446–448.)* The increase in blood flow through the pulmonary circulation during exercise increases the diameter of the pulmonary vessels and therefore decreases their resistance. The decrease in resistance can occur because the pulmonary vessels are very compliant and are large enough to prevent an increase in pulmonary artery blood pressure when cardiac output increases. The increased blood flow to the lung evens out the V/Q ratio, decreasing it at the top of the lung and increasing it at the bottom. Making the V/Q ratio more similar throughout the lung may decrease some of the shunting effect that normally occurs at the base of the lung where the V/Q ratio is quite low and may actually increase the oxygen saturation of arterial blood. The increased blood flow will also increase the surface area for respiratory exchange and therefore increase the diffusing capacity.

280. The answer is c. (*Boron, pp 705–711.*) Capillary blood draining from areas of the lung with low V/Q ratios has low oxygen saturations. Capillary blood draining from areas of the lung with high V/Q ratios does not have oxygen saturations higher than normal because, under normal circumstances, the blood is fully saturated. When blood from areas of low V/Q ratios (with less-than-normal saturations) combines with blood from high V/Q ratios (with no-more-than-normal saturations), the saturation of the combined blood is less than normal. The low saturation of the blood causes the P_{O_2} of the arterial blood to be lower than normal. In the lungs, the alveolar oxygen tension is higher in areas of high V/Q ratio and lower in areas of low V/Q ratio. When the air from the two lung regions combines, it produces a normal $P_{A_{O_2}}$. Because the alveolar P_{O_2} is normal and the arterial P_{O_2} is less than normal, the A – a gradient is greater than normal.

281. The answer is d. (*Boron, pp 669–673.*) In a normal person, there is an A - a gradient for O_2 of about 4 to 10 mmHg. The V/Q ratios at the apices of the lungs are greater than at the bases of the lungs; this results in end-pulmonary capillary blood coming from the apices with higher P_{O_2} and from the bases with lower P_{O_2} than normal. The P_{O_2} of the mixed blood from these areas must be determined by the average of their O_2 contents. Because of the nonlinearity of the oxyhemoglobin dissociation curve, the resultant Pa_{O_2} is not the average of the end-pulmonary capillary P_{O_2} values. In addition, about 2 to 5% of the blood returning to the left heart—that is, blood from the bronchial veins and from the thebesian veins draining the left ventricle—is venous blood that has not been oxygenated and constitutes a right-to-left absolute shunt. Normally, levels of alveolar and end-pulmonary capillary blood P_{O_2} do come into equilibrium. If they do not, as in some disease states, this alveolar-capillary block would contribute to the A – a gradient for O_2.

282. The answer is c. (*Boron, pp 618–621.*) Surfactant acts to diminish the surface tension of the lung. In the absence of surfactant, the lungs are more difficult to expand. Patients with a restrictive lung disease cannot expand their lungs as easily as normal, and, therefore, their total lung capacity is lower than normal. Because they have a lower total lung volume, the amount of gas they can exhale in 1 s (the FEV_1) is less than normal. Similarly, their forced vital capacity (FVC) is lower than normal. However, because they have a greater-than-normal recoil force, they can exhale a normal or a greater than normal fraction of their TLC in 1 s. Therefore, their FEV_1/FVC is normal or even slightly higher than normal. The greater recoil reduces the amount of gas they can inhale with each breath so their maximum voluntary ventilation (MVV) is less than normal.

283. The answer is a. *(Boron, pp 604–605, 867.)* The lung has many metabolic functions, including synthesis of surfactant and prostaglandins and withdrawal of prostaglandins and bradykinin from the circulation. Other metabolic functions include activation of angiotensin I to angiotensin II, release of histamine, and inactivation of serotonin. Prostaglandins E and F both are synthesized and removed from the circulation by the lungs.

284. The answer is d. *(Boron, pp 1262–1265. Guyton, pp 496–500.)* Hyperventilation occurs as soon as a person is exposed to low atmospheric pressures at high altitudes. The rise in pH attenuates the chemoreceptor response to low oxygen tensions. When the pH of the cerebrospinal fluid returns to normal, the chemoreceptors are restored to their normal responsiveness, and they are able to produce an even greater increase in ventilation. The plasma concentration of 2,3-DPG and, therefore, the oxygen-carrying capacity of hemoglobin increase with prolonged exposure to high altitudes. These changes increase the ability of the cardiovascular system to deliver oxygen to the tissues.

285. The answer is e. *(Boron, pp 656–661. Guyton, pp 390–391, 491.)* Cyanosis is the blue color of the skin produced by desaturated hemoglobin. Cyanosis appears when 5 g of hemoglobin per 100 mL of blood are desaturated. For a person with a normal hemoglobin concentration of 15 g/100 mL, cyanosis appears when one-third of the blood is desaturated. For a person with polycythemia (a higher-than-normal concentration of hemoglobin), cyanosis may appear when only one-fourth of the hemoglobin is desaturated. This individual may not be hypoxic because of the high concentration of saturated hemoglobin. On the other hand, a person with anemia (a lower than normal concentration of hemoglobin) may have a significant portion of the hemoglobin desaturated without displaying cyanosis. This individual will not appear cyanotic but may be hypoxic.

286. The answer is d. *(Boron, pp 674–684.)* A diffusion-limited transport process is one in which the alveolar gas does not reach equilibrium with the end-pulmonary capillary blood. When diffusional equilibrium does not occur, the amount of gas transferred is proportional to the concentration gradient and the permeability of the gas to the alveolar-capillary interface. Carbon monoxide (CO) is transported by a diffusion-limited process because it is avidly bound to hemoglobin. So much CO binds to hemoglobin that the partial pressure of CO in the capillary blood remains near zero. As a result, the concentration gradient from alveolar gas to capillary blood remains constant and the amount of CO diffusing across the alveolar-capillary interface depends only on the permeability of the gas. In contrast, all of the other gases reach equilibrium with the capillary blood, and, therefore, the amount of those gases that diffuses across the alveolar-capillary membrane is dependent on the amount of blood passing through the pulmonary capillaries. This type of transport process is described as perfusion-limited.

287. The answer is a. *(Boron, pp 1181–1182.)* Hyperventilation occurs when the rate of alveolar ventilation reduces the arterial P_{CO_2} below 40 mmHg. Pregnancy produces hyperventilation because progesterone stimulates the brainstem respiratory centers to increase alveolar ventilation above that required to maintain arterial P_{CO_2} at 40 mmHg. Sleep and morphine depress the respiratory centers and, therefore, produce hypoventilation (an arterial P_{CO_2} below 40 mmHg). During exercise, ventilation increases in parallel with carbon dioxide production so that the arterial P_{CO_2} remains at 40 mmHg. Metabolic alkalosis causes a small decrease in alveolar ventilation, producing a compensatory respiratory acidosis.

288. The answer is a. *(Boron, pp 1262–1265. Guyton, pp 496–500.)* Breathing air with a low partial pressure of oxygen will stimulate the peripheral chemoreceptors, which in turn will stimulate respiration. The increased alveolar ventilation will decrease the arterial P_{CO_2} to a value below normal (less than 40 mmHg). Although the increased ventilation will increase the arterial P_{O_2}, the resulting value will remain below normal for as long as the individual is breathing air with a low partial pressure of oxygen. A lower-than-normal arterial O_2 tension and a normal or greater-than-normal arterial CO_2 tension is usually a sign of a depressed respiratory center. A greater-than-normal arterial O_2 tension and a lower than normal arterial CO_2 tension can only occur if the person is breathing air with a greater-than-normal concentration of oxygen.

289. The answer is a. *(Boron, pp 559–562.)* Hyperventilation, by definition, reduces the arterial P_{CO_2} below normal, that is, to a value less than 40 mmHg. Low arterial P_{CO_2} in the blood perfusing the brain causes vasoconstriction of the cerebral vasculature, leading to a lowering of blood flow to the brain. The low arterial CO_2 will increase the pH of the arterial blood (i.e., produce a respiratory alkalosis) and decrease the activity of the central chemoreceptors. Pulmonary vasculature, unlike the systemic vasculature, is dilated by low P_{CO_2} and high P_{O_2} and constricted by high P_{CO_2} and low P_{O_2}. The respiratory alkalosis will cause Ca^{2+} to bind to plasma proteins, lowering the concentration of ionized Ca^{2+}. Low concentrations of ionized Ca^{2+} increase the excitability of nerve and muscle membranes, causing them to contract spontaneously or with minimal stimulation. The increased contractile activity of skeletal muscle produced by low concentration of ionized Ca^{2+} is called tetany.

290. The answer is a. *(Boron, pp 693–694, 707–711.)* Patients with chronic lung disease typically have difficulty maintaining a normal arterial oxygen tension due to an increase in lung compliance and V/Q abnormalities. "Blue bloaters" are patients with cyanosis and peripheral edema. These patients have extensive areas of lung tissue with lower-than-normal V/Q ratios; therefore, they are not able to fully oxygenate their blood and then develop cyanosis. The low oxygen tension leads to increased pulmonary arterial resistance and enlarged right ventricles (cor pulmonale). The resulting increased central venous pressure causes peripheral edema (bloating). "Pink puffers" are able to maintain normal arterial P_{O_2} levels. All patients with chronic lung disease will have decreased vital capacity and expiratory flow rates and increased airway resistance.

291–292. The answers are 291-a, 292-c. *(Boron, pp 656–663.)* The oxyhemoglobin saturation (Hb O_2) curve represents the relationship between the partial pressure of oxygen and the amount of oxygen bound to hemoglobin (Hb). Normal Hb is 50% saturated with a P_{O_2} of approximately 27 mmHg (the P_{50}), 75% saturated with a P_{O_2} of 40 mmHg (the normal P_{O_2} of mixed venous blood), and almost 100% saturated at a P_{O_2} of 100 mmHg (the normal arterial P_{O_2}). Increasing the affinity of Hb for O_2 shifts the Hb

O_2 saturation curve to the left and decreases the P_{50}; decreasing the affinity of Hb for O_2 shifts the Hb O_2 saturation curve to the right and increases the P_{50}. Fetal blood has a higher-than-normal oxygen affinity and therefore is represented by the curve labeled **A.** Carbon monoxide (CO) competitively inhibits the binding of O_2 to Hb, so the total amount of O_2 that can bind to Hb at any PO_2 is less than normal. However, somewhat paradoxically, CO increases the affinity of Hb for O_2 so the HB O_2 curve is shifted to the left. The HB O_2 curve for blood exposed to CO is represented by the curve labeled **C,** which is shifted to the left but is unable to bind as much O_2 as normal at a PO_2 of 100 mmHg.

293–294. The answers are 293-e, 294-b. (*Boron, pp 545–546, 729–731.*) The low oxygen tension will stimulate the peripheral chemoreceptors, which will increase alveolar ventilation and decrease arterial CO_2 tension. The pulmonary congestion may be due to left heart failure, which will cause an increase in left atrial pressure and pulmonary artery pressure. The A – a gradient will be above normal because the average alveolar oxygen tension is somewhat above normal due to the hyperventilation and the blood analysis reveals a lower-than-normal arterial oxygen tension. Pulmonary arterial resistance will be increased due to the low oxygen tension. Providing oxygen to the patient increases the arterial O_2 tension and allows pulmonary vascular resistance to return to normal. Once arterial oxygen tension returns to normal, alveolar ventilation will no longer be stimulated and alveolar carbon dioxide tension and arterial H^+ ion concentration will both increase toward normal. Alveolar oxygen tension ($P_{A}O_2$) will increase because the patient is breathing gas with a high partial pressure of oxygen Even though the arterial PO_2 has increased, the high percent of oxygen in the inspired air will cause a much larger increase in alveolar oxygen tension, causing a further increase in the A – a gradient.

295–296. The answers are 295-e, 296-d. (*Boron, pp 704–711.*) A large intrapulmonary shunt will cause arterial oxygen tension to decrease. This will increase respiratory drive, causing a respiratory alkalosis, which will result in a low PCO_2 and a high pH. The low oxygen tension may also produce a lactic acidosis, which may attenuate the rise in pH produced by hyperventilation. A patient with metabolic acidosis will have a lower-than-normal pH, which will stimulate the chemical and peripheral chemoreceptors. The ensuing rise in alveolar ventilation will lower PCO_2 and slightly increase PO_2.

297. The answer is e. *(Boron, pp 606–616, 678–682, 710.)* The reduced lung volumes indicate a restrictive lung disease. Although the amount of gas that can be expelled from the lung in 1 s will be less than normal, the increased recoil force of the lung will produce an FEV_1/FVC ratio that is close to normal. Patients with restrictive lung disease have small tidal volumes. The diffusing capacity will be reduced because the small lung volumes reduce the surface area available for gas exchange. The presence of V/Q abnormalities is indicated by the need for supplemental oxygen.

298. The answer is b. *(Boron, pp 621–632.)* Most of the airway is within the thoracic cavity, and, therefore, the intrathoracic pressure affects airway diameter and resistance. The intrathoracic pressure is most negative at the total lung capacity. The negative thoracic pressure increases airway diameter and decreases airway resistance. During a forced expiration or at the residual volume, the intrathoracic pressure is positive, compressing the airways and increasing their resistance. The vagus nerve constricts airway smooth muscle. Low oxygen will have little effect on airway tone.

Renal and Acid-Base Physiology

Questions

DIRECTIONS: Each question below contains several suggested responses. Select the **one best** response to each question.

299. The consumption of oxygen by the kidney

a. Decreases as blood flow increases
b. Is regulated by erythropoietin
c. Remains constant as blood flow increases
d. Directly reflects the level of sodium transport
e. Is greatest in the medulla

300. A 49-year-old man is brought to the emergency room with severe gastric pain after ingesting a large quantity of unknown fluid. Laboratory results show the following:

plasma pH   = 7.03
bicarbonate   = 12 meq/L
potassium   = 6.3 mM
anion gap   = 32 meq/L
ionized calcium = 1 mM

His blood pressure is 80/40 mmHg and his pulse rate is 102 beats/min. The ECG shows sinus tachycardia and peaked T waves. The high anion gap is most likely caused by a higher-than-normal plasma concentration of which of the following?

a. Lactate
b. Potassium
c. Chloride
d. Bicarbonate
e. Citrate

Questions 301–302

301. A 65-year-old man with uncontrolled type II diabetes and sustained hyperglycemia (serum glucose = 550 mg/dL) and polyuria (5 L/day) is evaluated in the hospital's clinical laboratory because his urine glucose concentration (<100 mM) was much lower than expected. The graph below illustrates the relationship between plasma glucose concentration and renal glucose reabsorption for this patient. The GFR is 100 mL/min. Which of the following is the renal threshold for glucose?

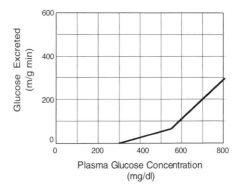

a. 50 mg/dL
b. 100 mg/dL
c. 200 mg/dL
d. 300 mg/dL
e. 400 mg/dL

302. Which of the following is the T_{max} for glucose?

a. 100 mg/min
b. 200 mg/min
c. 300 mg/min
d. 400 mg/min
e. 500 mg/min

303. In the presence of antidiuretic hormone (ADH), the filtrate will be isotonic to plasma in which of the following?

a. Descending limb of the loop of Henle
b. Ascending limb of the loop of Henle
c. Cortical collecting tubule
d. Medullary collecting tubule
e. Renal pelvis

304. A 16-year-old girl with hypertension, hypervolemia, and hypokalemic metabolic alkalosis is diagnosed with Liddle's syndrome when a blood test reveals low plasma aldosterone levels. The administration of triamterene (a sodium channel antagonist) reverses her clinical condition. Which of the following is the major defect in Liddle's syndrome?

a. An increased sodium reabsorption by the distal nephron
b. An increase in renin secretion by the juxtaglomerular apparatus
c. An inability of the distal nephron to secrete potassium
d. An inability of the distal nephron to secrete hydrogen
e. An inability of the distal nephron to concentrate urine

305. A 10-month-old well-nourished, lethargic infant is brought to the emergency room with a history of profuse watery diarrhea for 5 days. His mother reports that he had a marked decrease in urine output and continuous vomiting. Serum sodium is 190 mmol/L; urine sodium is 18 mmol/L. The infant is treated for gastroenteritis and a saline drip is started. After 3 days, he appears well and alert and his diarrhea and vomiting have subsided. However, he still has hypernatremia, polyuria, and low urine sodium. His persistent clinical signs are most likely due to which of the following?

a. Hyperaldosteronism
b. Diabetes insipidus
c. Diabetes mellitus
d. Renal failure
e. Hypothyroidism

306. A previously well 18-year-old girl is admitted to the ICU because of altered mental status. She does not respond to instructions and her arms are postured in a flexor position. Laboratory data reveal a serum sodium concentration of 125 mmol/L. Her friends indicate that the patient had taken ecstasy at a party the night before, and because she was extremely thirsty the next morning, she had consumed a lot of water in a short period of time. Assuming that the reduction in osmolarity is entirely due to water consumption and that her initial weight was 60 kg, approximately how much water would she have had to drink to produce the observed hyponatremia?

a. 5 L
b. 6 L
c. 7 L
d. 8 L
e. 9 L

307. A previously well 12-year-old boy is brought to the emergency room with vomiting and severe abdominal cramps after a prolonged period of exercise. Laboratory findings (high serum creatinine and urea) suggest acute renal failure. Following treatment and recovery, his serum uric acid concentration (0.6 mg/dL) remains consistently below normal. To determine if his low serum uric acid level is related to renal dysfunction, uric acid clearance studies are conducted and the following data are obtained:

Urine volume   = 1 mL/min
Urine uric acid = 36 mg/dL

What is the patient's uric acid clearance?

a. 6 mL/min
b. 12 mL/min
c. 24 mL/min
d. 48 mL/min
e. 60 mL/min

308. Renin secretion by the kidney is increased by which of the following?

a. Increasing mean blood pressure
b. Increasing glomerular filtration rate
c. Increasing sympathetic nerve activity
d. Increasing angiotensin II synthesis
e. Increasing atrial natriuretic peptide secretion

309. Na$^+$ is reabsorbed from the basolateral surface of the renal epithelial cells by which of the following?

a. Na/H exchange
b. Na-glucose cotransport
c. Na-K pump
d. Facilitated diffusion
e. Solvent drag

310. Which of the following is most likely to cause an increase in the glomerular filtration rate?

a. Contraction of mesangial cells
b. Blockage of the ureter
c. Release of renin from the juxtaglomerular apparatus
d. Dilation of the afferent arterioles
e. Volume depletion

311. The daily production of hydrogen ion from CO_2 is primarily buffered by which of the following?

a. Extracellular bicarbonate
b. Red blood cell bicarbonate
c. Red blood cell hemoglobin
d. Plasma proteins
e. Plasma phosphate

312. Glomerular filtration rate would be decreased by which of the following?

a. Constriction of the efferent arteriole
b. An increase in afferent arteriolar pressure
c. Compression of the renal capsule
d. A decrease in the concentration of plasma protein
e. An increase in renal blood flow

313. A 19-year-old man is admitted to the hospital after ingesting antifreeze containing ethylene glycol. His blood test reveals the following: Na$^+$ = 135 mEq/L, K$^+$ = 5 mEq/L, Cl$^-$ = 100 mEq/L, HCO$_3^-$ = 5 mEq/L, BUN = 25 mg/dL, Cr = 1.7 mg/dL, ABG pH 7.13. What is the size of his anion gap?

a. 5 mEq/L
b. 10 mEq/L
c. 15 mEq/L
d. 25 mEq/L
e. 30 mEq/L

314. The secretion of H^+ in the proximal tubule is primarily associated with which of the following?

a. Excretion of potassium ion
b. Excretion of hydrogen ion
c. Reabsorption of calcium ion
d. Reabsorption of bicarbonate ion
e. Reabsorption of phosphate ion

Questions 315–316

315. A 32-year-old man complaining of fatigue and muscle weakness is seen by his physician. He has a prominent forehead, protruding jaw, widely spaced teeth, and a large nose. Blood tests reveal a serum glucose level of 325 mg/dL and serum creatinine of 0.8 mg/dL. Results of a 24-h urine analysis are as follows:

Total volume = 5 L
Total glucose = 375 g
Total creatinine = 2.4 g

Which of the following is this patient's approximate glomerular filtration rate?

a. 75 mL/min
b. 100 mL/min
c. 125 mL/min
d. 200 mL/min
e. 275 mL/min

316. Approximately how much glucose is reabsorbed by this patient's kidneys?

a. 225 g/day
b. 300 g/day
c. 375 g/day
d. 450 g/day
e. 600 g/day

317. A 40-year-old woman is admitted to the intensive care unit with hypotension and shortness of breath. Arterial blood gases reveal: Pa_{CO_2}, 10 mmHg, and bicarbonate, 12 meq/L. What is her acid-base status?

a. Normal
b. Respiratory acidosis
c. Metabolic acidosis
d. Respiratory alkalosis
e. Metabolic alkalosis

318. A 56-year-old man is admitted to the emergency room after ingesting a large dose of aspirin, most of which is still within the vascular system. The patient is diaphoretic and tachypneic and has the following blood gases: pH of 7.5, P_{CO_2} of 17 mmHg, and bicarbonate of 13 mmol/L.

Aspirin has a pK of 3.5 and when it is in the un-ionized state will rapidly cross the blood-brain barrier. Which of the following treatment options would be most deleterious to this patient?

a. Breathing supplemental oxygen
b. Infusing bicarbonate
c. Decreasing alveolar ventilation
d. Increasing fluid volume
e. Administering activated charcoal

319. A 38-year-old woman is admitted to the hospital by her physician because of decreased urine output. Prior to admission she was rehearsing for a dance performance and had been taking Motrin for pain. Laboratory data reveal: blood urea nitrogen, 49 mg/dL; serum sodium, 135 mmol/L; serum creatinine, 7.5 mg/dL; urine sodium, 33 mmol/L, and urine creatinine, 90 mg/dL. Her fractional sodium excretion is approximately

a. 0.5%
b. 1.0%
c. 1.5%
d. 2.0%
e. 3.0%

320. Use the following laboratory values to calculate the net acid excretion:

Plasma pH   = 7.2
Urine flow   = 1.2 L/day
Urine bicarbonate   = 2 meq/L
Urine titratable acids = 24 meq/L
Urine ammonium   = 38 meq/L
Urine pH   = 5.4

a. 60 meq/L
b. 64 meq/L
c. 68 meq/L
d. 72 meq/L
e. 76 meq/L

321. Use the following laboratory data to estimate the renal blood flow:

Renal artery PAH = 6 mg/dL
Renal vein PAH = 0.6 mg/dL
Urinary PAH   = 25 mg/mL
Urine flow   = 1.5 ml/min

Renal plasma flow is approximately

a. 475 mL/min
b. 550 mL/min
c. 625 mL/min
d. 700 mL/min
e. 775 mL/min

322. If a substance appears in the renal artery but not in the renal vein,

a. Its clearance is equal to the glomerular filtration rate
b. It must be reabsorbed by the kidney
c. Its urinary concentration must be higher than its plasma concentration
d. Its clearance is equal to the renal plasma flow
e. It must be filtered by the kidney

323. A freely filterable substance that is neither reabsorbed nor secreted has a renal artery concentration of 12 mg/mL and a renal vein concentration of 9 mg/mL. Which of the following is the filtration fraction (GFR/RPF)?

a. 0.05
b. 0.15
c. 0.25
d. 0.35
e. 0.45

324. A 46-year-old man presents to his physician with a 12-week history of headaches. The headaches, mainly frontal, are worse in the morning and have begun to wake him at night. A trans-sphenoidal biopsy shows a non-infectious, chronic inflammatory process that is diagnosed as neurohypophysitis (an inflammation of the neurohypophysis). Which one of the following best describes his urine?

a. A higher-than-normal flow of hypotonic urine
b. A higher-than-normal flow of hypertonic urine
c. A normal flow of hypertonic urine
d. A lower-than-normal flow of hypotonic urine
e. A lower-than-normal flow of hypertonic urine

325. A 29-year-old woman is admitted to the hospital because of increasing dyspnea and sudden swelling of both feet. An examination of her chest shows a severe pectus excavatum with only 2 cm of space between the vertebral bodies and the sternum. Pulmonary function tests show FVC and FEV_1/FVC values that were 15 and 100%, respectively, of predicted. Which of the following laboratory measurements will most likely be below normal in this patient?

a. Alveolar-arterial gradient
b. Arterial P_{CO_2}
c. Hemoglobin concentration
d. Plasma bicarbonate concentration
e. Arterial pH

326. The pH of the tubular fluid in the distal nephron can be lower than that in the proximal tubule because

a. A greater sodium gradient can be established across the wall of the distal nephron than across the wall of the proximal tubule
b. More buffer is present in the tubular fluid of the distal nephron than in the proximal tubule
c. More hydrogen ion is secreted into the distal nephron than into the proximal tubule
d. The brush border of the distal nephron contains more carbonic anhydrase than that of the proximal tubule
e. The tight junctions of the distal nephron are less leaky to solute than those of the proximal tubule

327. Which of the following statements about renin is true?

a. It is secreted by cells of the proximal tubule
b. Its secretion leads to loss of sodium and water from plasma
c. Its secretion is stimulated by increased mean renal arterial pressure
d. It converts angiotensinogen to angiotensin I
e. It converts angiotensin I to angiotensin II

328. A 63-year-old woman is brought to the emergency room complaining of fatigue and headaches. She appears confused and apathetic. She has been taking diuretics to treat her hypertension and paroxetine for her depression. Laboratory results are as follows:

urine flow: 1.9 L/day
serum sodium: 125 mmol/L
serum potassium: 4 mmol/L
urine osmolality: 385 mOsm/L
urine sodium: 125 mmol/L
urine potassium: 25 mmol/L

Which of the following is this patient's approximate free water clearance?

a. −0.20 L/day
b. −0.50/day
c. −0.75/day
d. +0.2/day
e. +0.50/day

329. A 28-year-old woman is brought to the emergency room after developing hypokalemic paralysis. Arterial blood gas analysis shows a PaO_2 of 102 mmHg and a pH of 7.1. She is diagnosed with type I renal tubular acidosis caused by Sjögren's syndrome (an autoimmune tubulointerstitial nephropathy that damages the H^+-ATPase on the distal nephron). Which of the following laboratory measurements will most likely be normal in this patient?

a. Net acid excretion
b. Aldosterone secretion
c. Serum bicarbonate
d. Urine ammonium
e. Anion gap

330. The effective renal plasma flow, which equals the clearance of PAH, is less than the true renal plasma flow because

a. The fraction of PAH filtered is less than the filtration fraction
b. The plasma entering the renal vein contains a small amount of PAH
c. The cortical and medullary collecting ducts are able to reabsorb some PAH
d. The calculated clearance of PAH depends on the urinary flow rate
e. The measured value of the plasma PAH concentration is less than the actual PAH concentration

331. Most of the glucose that is filtered through the glomerulus undergoes reabsorption in which of the following?

a. Proximal tubule
b. Descending limb of the loop of Henle
c. Ascending limb of the loop of Henle
d. Distal tubule
e. Collecting duct

332. Which of the following structural features distinguishes the epithelial cells of the proximal tubule from those of the distal tubule?

a. The distal tubule has a thicker basement membrane
b. The proximal tubule has a thicker basement membrane
c. The proximal tubule has a more extensive brush border
d. The proximal tubule forms the juxtaglomerular apparatus
e. The distal tubule has fewer tight intercellular junctions

333. Which of the following statements concerning the renal handling of proteins is correct?

a. Proteins are more likely to be filtered if they are negatively charged than if they are uncharged
b. Proteins can be filtered and secreted but not reabsorbed by the kidney
c. Most of the protein excreted each day is derived from tubular secretion
d. Protein excretion is directly related to plasma protein concentration
e. Protein excretion is increased by sympathetic stimulation of the kidney

334. Glomerular filtration rate (GFR) and renal blood flow (RBF) will both be increased if

a. The efferent and afferent arterioles are both dilated
b. The efferent and afferent arterioles are both constricted
c. Only the afferent arteriole is constricted
d. Only the efferent arteriole is constricted
e. The afferent arteriole is constricted and the efferent arteriole is dilated

335. A 23-year-old man is brought to the emergency room after collapsing during basketball practice. On admission he is lethargic and appears confused. His coach reports that he was drinking a lot of water during practice. His symptoms are most likely caused by increased

a. Intracellular tonicity
b. Extracellular tonicity
c. Extracellular volume
d. Intracellular volume
e. Plasma volume

336. Which one of the following statements about ammonia (NH_3) is correct?

a. It is impermeable to the epithelial cells of the proximal tubule
b. It is classified as a titratable acid
c. It is produced by epithelial cells in the distal nephron
d. It reduces the concentration of bicarbonate in the plasma
e. Its synthesis is increased in respiratory acidosis

337. The amount of potassium excreted by the kidney will decrease if

a. Distal tubular flow increases
b. Circulating aldosterone levels increase
c. Dietary intake of potassium increases
d. Na^+ reabsorption by the distal nephron decreases
e. The excretion of organic ions decreases

338. A respiratory acidosis that results in an increase in the concentration of hydrogen ion in arterial blood from 40 meq/L (pH 7.4) to 50 meq/L (pH 7.3) would

a. Stimulate the peripheral chemoreceptors
b. Decrease the amount of ammonium excreted in the urine
c. Inhibit the central chemoreceptors
d. Increase the pH of the urine
e. Decrease the concentration of HCO_3^- in arterial blood

339. Which of the following substances will be more concentrated at the end of the proximal tubule than at the beginning of the proximal tubule?

a. Glucose
b. Creatinine
c. Sodium
d. Bicarbonate
e. Phosphate

340. When a person is dehydrated, hypotonic fluid will be found in which of the following?

a. Glomerular filtrate
b. Proximal tubule
c. Loop of Henle
d. Cortical collecting tubule
e. Distal collecting duct

341. Electrically neutral active transport of sodium and chloride from the lumen of the kidney occurs in which of the following?

a. Proximal tubule
b. Descending limb of the loop of Henle
c. Thin ascending limb of the loop of Henle
d. Cortical collecting duct
e. Medullary collecting duct

342. A 65-year-old man is admitted to the hospital because of profound muscle weakness. His blood glucose is 485 mg/dL and his serum potassium is 8.2 mmol/L. He is diagnosed with diabetic ketoacidosis and hyperkalemia. In addition to the serum glucose and potassium, which one of the following laboratory values would most likely be above normal?

a. Serum HCO_3^-
b. Anion gap
c. Arterial P_{CO_2}
d. Plasma pH
e. Blood volume

343. Decreasing the resistance of the afferent arteriole in the glomerulus of the kidney will decrease which of the following?

a. The renal plasma flow
b. The filtration fraction
c. The oncotic pressure of the peritubular capillary blood
d. The glomerular filtration rate
e. None of the above

344. If GFR increases, proximal tubular reabsorption of salt and water will increase by a process called glomerulotubular balance. Contributions to this process include which of the following?

a. An increase in peritubular capillary hydrostatic pressure
b. A decrease in peritubular sodium concentration
c. An increase in peritubular oncotic pressure
d. An increase in proximal tubular flow
e. An increase in peritubular capillary flow

345. Renin release from the juxtaglomerular apparatus is inhibited by which of the following?

a. Beta-adrenergic agonists
b. Prostaglandins
c. Aldosterone
d. Stimulation of the macula densa
e. Increased pressure within the afferent arterioles

346. A 24-year-old man with a history of renal insufficiency is admitted to the hospital after taking a large amount of ibuprofen. His BUN is 150 mg/dL. This patient's high serum urea nitrogen was most likely caused by which of the following?

a. An increased synthesis of urea by the liver
b. An increased reabsorption of urea by the proximal tubules
c. A decreased secretion of urea by the distal tubules
d. A decreased glomerular filtration rate
e. An increased renal blood flow

347. Which one of the following statements about aldosterone is correct?

a. It produces its effect by activating cAMP
b. It produces its effect by increasing distal tubular permeability to sodium
c. It causes an increased reabsorption of hydrogen ion
d. It has its main effect on the proximal tubule
e. It is secreted in response to an increase in blood pressure

348. Which of the following is the effect of antidiuretic hormone (ADH) on the kidney?

a. Increased permeability of the distal nephron to water
b. Increased glomerular filtration rate
c. Increased excretion of Na^+
d. Increased excretion of water
e. Increased diameter of the renal artery

349. A 65-year-old man with type I diabetes presents to the emergency room with impaired mental status and generalized muscle weakness. Laboratory tests reveal a blood glucose of 500 mg/dL, a potassium concentration of 8.3 mmol/L, an anion gap of 22 mmol/L, a P_{CO_2} of 50 mmHg, and a bicarbonate of 14 mmol/L Which of the following blood values is atypical?

a. Hyperglycemia
b. Hyperkalemia
c. High anion gap
d. Hypercapnia
e. High creatinine

350. The ability of the kidney to excrete concentrated urine will increase if

a. The reabsorption of Na^+ by the proximal tubule decreases
b. The flow of filtrate through the loop of Henle increases
c. The glomerular capillary pressure increases
d. The activity of the Na-K pump in the loop of Henle increases
e. The permeability of the collecting duct to water decreases

351. A 16-year-old pregnant girl is admitted to the hospital in labor. Her blood pressure is 130/85 mmHg and her plasma creatinine is 2.7 mg/dL (normal 0.6 to 1.2 mg/dL). Renal ultrasonography demonstrates severe bilateral hydronephrosis (enlarged kidney). Which of the following is the most likely cause of this patient's high creatinine levels?

a. Increased sympathetic nerve activity
b. Coarctation of the renal artery
c. Hyperproteinemia
d. Uretal obstruction
e. Hypovolemia

352. A 23-year-old girl is admitted to the hospital with a 3-month history of malaise and generalized muscle cramps. Laboratory results reveal: serum sodium of 144 mmol/L, serum potassium of 2.0 mmol/L, serum bicarbonate of 40 mmol/L, and arterial pH of 7.5. Which of the following is the most likely cause of this patient's hypokalemic alkalemia?

a. Hyperaldosteronism
b. Hyperventilation
c. Persistent diarrhea
d. Renal failure
e. Diabetes

353. The syndrome of inappropriate antidiuretic hormone secretion (SIADH) is caused by the excess release of ADH. SIADH will cause an increase in which of the following?

a. Concentration of plasma sodium
b. Intracellular volume
c. Urinary flow
d. Plasma oncotic pressure
e. Plasma osmolarity

354. Which one of the following comparisons between the distal nephron and the proximal tubule is correct?

a. The distal nephron is more permeable to hydrogen ion than the proximal tubule
b. The distal nephron is less responsive to aldosterone than the proximal tubule
c. The distal nephron has a more negative intraluminal potential than the proximal tubule
d. The distal nephron secretes less potassium than does the proximal tubule
e. The distal nephron secretes more hydrogen ion than does the proximal tubule

355. An increase in the concentration of NaCl in the intraluminal fluid with the ascending limb of the loop of Henle causes the macula densa to release which of the following?

a. ADH
b. Aldosterone
c. Adenosine
d. Renin
e. Angiotensinogen

356. Metabolic acidosis is caused by which of the following?

a. Hypoaldosteronism
b. Hyperventilation
c. Hypokalemia
d. Hypovolemia
e. Hypercalcemia

357. Aldosterone secretion is increased when there is an increase in the plasma concentration of which of the following?

a. ACTH
b. Chloride
c. Sodium
d. Hydrogen
e. Potassium

358. In which one of the following situations is urinary flow less than normal?

a. Diabetes insipidus
b. Diabetes mellitus
c. Sympathetic stimulation
d. Increased renal arterial pressure
e. Infusion of mannitol

359. Most of the volatile acid entering the blood is buffered by which of the following?

a. Bicarbonate
b. Plasma proteins
c. Hemoglobin
d. Phosphates
e. Lactate

360. Potassium-sparing diuretics inhibit Na^+ reabsorption in which of the following?

a. Proximal tubule
b. Thin descending limb of Henle's loop
c. Thick descending limb of Henle's loop
d. Distal convoluted tubule
e. Cortical collecting duct

361. Which of the following values will most likely be above normal in a diabetic patient with a blood glucose concentration of 600 mEq/L?

a. Urine flow
b. Intracellular volume
c. Plasma sodium concentration
d. Arterial pH
e. Alveolar P_{CO_2}

362. Which of the following will most likely be increased in a patient suffering from persistent diarrhea?

a. The filtered load of HCO_3^-
b. The production of ammonia by the proximal tubule
c. H^+ secretion by the distal nephron
d. The anion gap
e. The production of new bicarbonate by the distal nephron

363. In addition to increasing the permeability of the collecting duct to water, ADH increases the permeability of the collecting duct to

a. Hydrogen
b. Ammonium
c. Potassium
d. Sodium
e. Urea

364. The filtration fraction is increased by which of the following?

a. Increasing renal blood flow
b. Increasing afferent arteriolar resistance
c. Increasing efferent arteriolar resistance
d. Increasing plasma oncotic pressure
e. Increasing the pressure within Bowman's capsule

365. Which one of the following conditions causes a higher-than-normal plasma bicarbonate concentration?

a. Volume depletion
b. Renal failure
c. Hypoxemia
d. Diarrhea
e. Hypoaldosteronism

366. Which one of the following substances causes renal blood flow to decrease?

a. Nitric oxide
b. Bradykinin
c. Prostaglandins
d. Adenosine
e. Dopamine

367. Diuretics, such as acetazolamide, which produce their effect by inhibiting carbonic anhydrase, inhibit the reabsorption of sodium in which of the following?

a. The proximal tubule
b. The thick ascending limb of Henle's loop
c. The distal convoluted tubule
d. The cortical collecting duct
e. The outer medullary collecting duct

368. The extracellular potassium of a hyperkalemic patient can be decreased by administering which of the following drugs?

a. Atropine
b. Epinephrine
c. Glucagon
d. Lactic acid
e. Isotonic saline

369. Which one of the following blood-gas values is consistent with metabolic acidosis?

	$Paco_2$ (mmHg)	HCO_3^- (mM)	pH
a.	25	30	7.7
b.	35	20	7.3
c.	40	25	7.4
d.	50	30	7.1
e.	60	20	7.1

370. Hyperkalemia may be observed in patients with which of the following?

a. Volume depletion
b. Diuretic therapy
c. Administration of insulin
d. Metabolic alkalosis
e. Stimulation of adrenal medulla

371. Which point on the graph below represents the blood-gas values obtained from a patient who has ascended to high altitude?

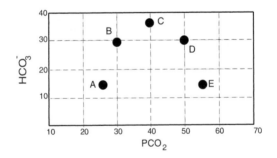

a. A
b. B
c. C
d. D
e. E

372. Which of the following substances is less concentrated at the end of the proximal tubule than at the beginning of the proximal tubule?

a. Creatinine
b. Hydrogen
c. Chloride
d. Phosphate
e. Sodium

373. What percentage of the filtered load of sodium is reabsorbed by the proximal tubule?

a. 15%
b. 25%
c. 45%
d. 65%
e. 95%

374. ANP (atrial natriuretic peptide) decreases Na reabsorption within which of the following?

a. The proximal tubule
b. The thick ascending limb of Henle's loop
c. The distal convoluted tubule
d. The cortical collecting duct
e. The inner medullary collecting duct

375. Free water clearance by the kidney is increased by which of the following?

a. Heart failure
b. Renal failure
c. Diuretic therapy
d. Diabetes mellitus
e. Diabetes insipidus

376. The renal clearance of phosphate is increased by which of the following hormones?

a. Aldosterone
b. Parathyroid hormone
c. Norepinephrine
d. Vasopressin
e. Angiotensin

377. Hyponatremia will result from an excess secretion of which of the following?

a. Vasopressin
b. Atrial natriuretic hormone
c. Norepinephrine
d. Insulin
e. Aldosterone

378. Which of the following will produce the greatest increase in potassium secretion?

a. A decrease in urinary flow rates
b. An increase in distal nephron sodium concentration
c. A decrease in circulating blood volume
d. An increase in sympathetic nerve activity
e. A decrease in renal blood flow

379. A decrease in the concentration of NaCl in the intraluminal fluid causes the juxtaglomerular apparatus to release which of the following hormones?

a. ADH
b. Aldosterone
c. Adenosine
d. Renin
e. Angiotensinogen

Questions 380–381

Use the following diagram of a nephron to answer the next two questions.

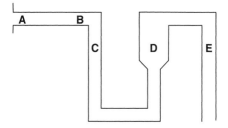

380. In the absence of ADH, the luminal Na^+ concentration is lowest at which of the following points?

a. A
b. B
c. C
d. D
e. E

381. Parathyroid hormone increases Ca^{2+} reabsorption at point

a. A
b. B
c. C
d. D
e. E

382. Aldosterone increases Na^+ reabsorption at point

a. A
b. B
c. C
d. D
e. E

383. Which of the following would be observed in a patient with chronic renal failure?

a. A decrease in the fractional excretion of sodium
b. An increase in the free water clearance
c. An increase in the anion gap
d. A decrease in the excretion of creatinine
e. An increase in the net acid excretion

384. The extracellular fluid volume of a normal individual is approximately

a. 5% of body mass
b. 10% of body mass
c. 20% of body mass
d. 40% of body mass
e. 60% of body mass

385. Which of the following signs of renal failure is caused by the loss of a hormone produced by the kidney?

a. Edema
b. Hypertension
c. Anemia
d. Uremia
e. Acidosis

386. A 39-year-old man presents to the emergency room complaining of tingling in his hands and muscle twitching. On admission, the patient is alert and stable, with an initial examination remarkable only for carpopedal spasm. Which of the following blood gas values will most likely be observed in this patient?

	$Paco_2$ (mM)	HCO_3^-
a.	50	40
b.	60	20
c.	40	30
d.	30	15
e.	20	20

Renal and Acid-Base Physiology

Answers

299. The answer is d. (*Boron, p 784. Guyton, p 369.*) In the kidney, oxygen is used primarily to support active transport of solutes, especially sodium, out of the tubules. In fact, oxygen consumption by the kidney is directly proportional to the amount of sodium reabsorbed and is greatest in the cortex, where most tubular reabsorption of sodium occurs. An increase in renal blood flow will raise the glomerular filtration rate and increase the quantity of solute to be transported, so that oxygen consumption increases as blood flow increases and the arteriovenous oxygen difference remains constant. This is in contrast to the situation in other organs where increases in blood flow are accompanied by a decrease in arteriovenous oxygen difference. Erythropoietin is released in response to renal hypoxia and acts to increase erythrocyte production.

300. The answer is e. (*Boron, pp 53–54. Guyton, pp 361–363.*) The anion gap is the difference between the concentration of Na^+ and the concentration of the major plasma anions, Cl^- and HCO_3^-. The minor ions, lactate, phosphate, and sulfate, comprise the anion gap. Increases in lactate or citrate could have produced the anion gap. The low calcium favors citrate as the cause of the anion gap because citrate complexes with calcium. The high serum potassium concentration accounts for the peaked T waves seen on the EKG. Acidosis caused the shift of K^+ from the intracellular to the extracellular space. The low calcium produced relaxation of vascular smooth muscle, accounting for the low blood pressure.

301–302. The answers are 301-d, 302-e. (*Guyton, pp 298–299.*) The renal threshold for glucose is the plasma concentration at which glucose first appears in the urine. The graph shows that glucose is excreted at a plasma concentration of 300 mg/dL. (This is higher than the typical value of 200 mg/dL.) Glucose appears in the urine at a filtered load less than the T_{max} for glucose because of the differences in the reabsorptive capacity of the nephrons. Some nephrons can only reabsorb a small amount of glucose. When their reabsorptive capacity is exceeded, glucose is excreted. Other nephrons can absorb much more glucose. The T_{max} represents the average reabsorptive capacity of all the renal nephrons. The T_{max} for glucose is the maximum rate of glucose reabsorption from the kidney. Typically, the T_{max} is 375 mg/min. However, the Tm in this patient is 500 mg/min. The higher-than-normal reabsorptive capacity accounts for the lower-than-expected urinary concentration. The Tm is calculated by subtracting the amount of glucose excreted from the filtered load at any plasma concentration at which the amount of glucose excreted increases linearly as plasma glucose concentration increases. For example, when the plasma glucose concentration is 600 mg/dL, the filtered load of glucose is 600 mg/min, the amount of glucose excreted is 100 mg/min, and the amount of glucose reabsorbed (the Tm) is 500 mg/min.

303. The answer is c. *(Boron, pp 830–831.)* In the absence of antidiuretic hormone (ADH, vasopressin), the cortical and medullary collecting tubules and ducts are impermeable to water. ADH increases the water permeability of these nephron segments and allows the filtrate to reach osmotic equilibrium with the interstitial fluid surrounding the nephron. The interstitial fluid in the cortex of the kidney is isotonic to plasma, and, therefore, the filtrate can become isotonic to plasma in the cortical collecting tubule. The interstitial fluid is hypertonic to plasma in the medullary collecting tubule, and so the filtrate becomes hypertonic to plasma in this region of the nephron and remains hypertonic as it passes through the renal pelvis. ADH has no effect on the water permeability of the loop of Henle. The filtrate is hypertonic to plasma in the descending limb and becomes hypotonic to plasma by the time it reaches the end of the ascending limb of the loop of Henle.

304. The answer is a. *(Boron, pp 786, 823–824. Guyton, pp 340–341, 369, 872–873.)* Sodium reabsorption in the distal nephron is normally under the control of aldosterone. In patients with Liddle's syndrome, an autosomal dominant form of hypertension accompanied by hypokalemia, metabolic alkalosis, and low plasma renin activity, the distal nephron Na^+ reabsorbs despite low levels of aldosterone and renin in the plasma. The alkalosis and hypokalemia are secondary to the increased sodium reabsorption. Liddle's syndrome resembles primary hyperaldosteronism and is difficult to diagnose.

305. The answer is b. *(Boron, pp 843–844.)* Diabetes insipidus is a disease caused by decreased release of ADH from the posterior pituitary or the inability of the kidney to response to ADH. It is characterized by high serum Na^+, polyuria, and low urine osmolarity. The low urine osmolarity in the presence of the volume depletion points to diabetes insipidus. The diagnosis is confirmed by the persistent polyuria and low urine sodium after the baby's volume is returned to normal.

306. The answer is a. *(Boraon, pp 50–53, 80–81. Guyton, pp 272–273.)* When water is ingested from the intestine, it enters the plasma and rapidly achieves osmotic equilibrium with the interstitial and intracellular compartments. A sodium concentration of 125 mM is equivalent to an osmolarity of 250 milliosmoles/L. Assuming that her normal osmolarity of 285 millimoles/L was reduced to 250 milliosmoles by the ingestion of water, she drank approximately 5 L. The amount of water ingested by the patient was not likely this high because she probably lost significant amount of salt as sweat while under the influence of ecstasy. Her signs and symptoms are due to the brain swelling caused by hypotonicity.

$$\text{Osmolarity} = \frac{\text{Milliosmoles}}{\text{Volume}}$$

$$250 \text{ milliosmoles/L} = \frac{60 \text{ kg} \times 60\% \times 284}{\text{Volume}}$$

$$\text{Total Volume} = \frac{10{,}224 \text{ milliosmoles}}{250 \text{ milliosmoles/L}} \approx 41 \text{ L}$$

$$\text{Volume Consumed} = \text{Total Volume} - \text{Original volume}$$

$$\text{Volume Consumed} = 41 \text{ L} - 36 \text{ L} = 5 \text{ L}$$

307. The answer is e. *(Boron, pp 801–802.)* Clearance is a measure of how much plasma is totally cleared of a substance. It is calculated using the formula

$$\text{Clearance} = \frac{U_{\text{uric acid}} \times \dot{V}}{P_{\text{uric acid}}} = \frac{36 \text{ mg/dL} \times 1 \text{ mL/min}}{0.6 \text{ mg/dL}} = 60 \text{ mL/min}$$

The boy's hypouricemia is an inherited defect in the ability to reabsorb uric acid by the anion/urate exchangers on proximal tubule cells rather than an increased secretion of uric acid. Patients with hypouricemia sometimes develop exercise-induced acute renal failure. Although the mechanism is not known, some investigators suggest that uric acid has an important antioxidant role in the kidney and that the oxygen radicals produced during prolonged exercise are responsible for the acute renal failure in patients with low uric acid levels.

308. The answer is c. (*Boron, pp 746–748, 866–867.*) Renin secretion is stimulated by the sympathetic nerves innervating the juxtaglomerular apparatus. Increasing mean blood pressure decreases sympathetic activity. Changes in GFR are detected by the macula densa. Decreases in GFR lead to an increase in renin release, whereas increases in GFR lead to the secretion of a mediator, perhaps adenosine or ATP, which contracts the afferent arteriole (tubuloglomerular feedback). ANP and angiotensin II will decrease renin release.

309. The answer is c. (*Boron, pp 774–779.*) The intracellular Na^+ concentration of renal epithelial cells is pumped out of renal epithelial cells by Na-K pumps located on the basolateral surface of the epithelial cells. The Na/H exchanger and the Na-glucose transporter are located on the apical surface of the epithelial cells. Na^+ is transported from the peritubular spaces to the capillaries by solvent drag.

310. The answer is d. (*Boron, pp 769–770. Guyton, pp 286–290.*) The GFR is proportional to the glomerular capillary hydrostatic pressure, the renal plasma flow, and the surface area and hydraulic conductivity of the diffusion barrier between the glomerular capillary and Bowman's space. Dilating the afferent arteriole causes an increase in glomerular capillary pressure and, therefore, an increase in GFR. Volume depletion causes a release of renin from the juxtaglomerular cells, leading to an increase in angiotensin II (AII) that causes constriction of the glomerular capillaries and contraction of the mesangial cells. Contraction of the mesangial cells causes a decrease in the surface area of the diffusion barrier between the glomerular capillary and Bowman's space. Blockage of the ureter causes an increase in tubular pressure that retards the filtration of water from the capillary to the nephron.

311. The answer is c. *(Boron, pp 642–646.)* Aerobic metabolism produces 13,000 to 24,000 mmol CO_2 per day. This yields close to that amount of H^+ ions produced per day via the reaction $CO_2 + H_2O \div H_2CO_3 \div H^+ + HCO_3^-$. At the tissues, CO_2 diffuses into the red blood cells, where the enzyme carbonic anhydrase accelerates the above reaction. The H^+ produced is buffered mainly by the large amount of hemoglobin in the red blood cells. Bicarbonate is not an effective buffer of volatile acid (from CO_2).

312. The answer is c. *(Boron, pp 764–765. Guyton, pp 286–288.)* Glomerular filtration rate (GFR) will decrease is there is a decrease in the net glomerular capillary pressure or the flow of fluid through the glomerulus. The net glomerular capillary pressure (for Starling forces) is equal to the glomerular capillary pressure minus the sum of the plasma oncotic pressure and intrarenal pressure. Compression of the renal capsule increases the intrarenal pressure and therefore decreases the net capillary filtration pressure. Constriction of the efferent arteriole increases glomerular capillary pressure. Decreasing the concentration of plasma protein will decrease the plasma oncotic pressure and lead to an increase in GFR.

313. The answer is e. *(Boron, pp 53–54. Guyton, pp 362–363.)* The anion gap is equal to the difference between the plasma concentration of sodium, the major cation in the plasma, and the sum of the concentrations of plasma chloride and bicarbonate, the major measured anions in the plasma.

$$\text{Anion gap} = [Na^+] - ([Cl^-] + [HCO_3^-])$$
$$= 135 \text{ mEq/L} - (100 \text{ mEq/L} + 5 \text{ mEq/L})$$
$$= 30 \text{ mEq/L}$$

The normal-plasma concentrations of Na^+, Cl^-, and HCO_3^- are 142, 105, and 24 mEq/L, respectively. The normal anion gap is from 8 to 16 mEq/L. The anion gap is elevated when the concentration of unmeasured anions in the plasma increases. For example, diabetic ketoacidosis and lactic acidosis produce an increased anion gap. A high anion gap metabolic acidosis is also caused by the metabolic byproducts (oxalic and glycolic acid) of ethylene glycol, a component of antifreeze.

314. The answer is d. *(Boron, 68–69, 776–777. Guyton, pp 353–354.)* In the proximal tubule, a large amount of H^+ ion is secreted into the tubule lumen via an Na^+-H^+ antiporter (exchanger). Most of this H^+ combines with bicarbonate ion in the tubular fluid to form CO_2 and water. The CO_2 diffuses into the proximal tubular cells, where the opposite reaction takes place to form H^+ and HCO_3^-. The HCO_3^- exits the cells on the basolateral side and enters the blood as reabsorbed bicarbonate. Carbonic anhydrase is located on the luminal surface of the cells as well as inside the cells to facilitate the above reactions.

315–316. The answers are 315-d, 316-e. (Boron, pp 748–749. Guyton, pp 309–312.) Glomerular filtration rate is determined approximately equal to the clearance of creatinine which in this case is

$$\text{Creatinine Clearance} = \frac{\text{Creatinine Excreted}}{\text{Plasma Creatinine Concentration}}$$

$$\text{Creatinine Clearance} = \frac{2.4 \text{ g/day}}{0.8 \text{ mg/dL}} = 300 \text{ L/day} = 208 \text{ mL/min}$$

The rate of glucose reabsorption is the difference between the glucose excreted and the glucose filtered, which is this case, is

$$\text{Glucose Reabsorbed} = \text{Glucose Filtered} - \text{Glucose Excreted}$$
$$\text{Filtered} = [G]_P \times \text{GFR} = 325 \text{ mg/dL} \times 208 \text{ mL/min} = 676 \text{ mL/min}$$
$$\text{Excreted} = 375 \text{ g/day} = 260 \text{ mg/min}$$
$$\text{Reabsorbed} = 676 \text{ mg/min} - 260 \text{ mg/min} = 416 \text{ mg/min} = 599 \text{ g/day}$$

This patient has the classic signs of hypersecretion of growth hormone in adults, including increased plasma glucose concentration. This disease, called acromegaly, occurs in adults after the epiphysis of the long bones has closed. Hypersecretion of growth hormone in children produce gigantism.

317. The answer is d. The arterial pH can be calculated using the Henderson-Hesselbach equation

$$pH = 6.1 + \log \frac{HCO_3^-}{0.03 \text{ mM/mmHg} \times P_{CO_2}}$$

$$pH = 6.1 + \log \frac{12 \text{ mM}}{0.03 \text{ mM/mmHg} \times 10 \text{ mmHg}}$$

$$pH = 6.1 + \log\frac{12}{0.3} = 6.1 + 1.6 = 7.7$$

The patient has an alkalemia, which is most likely due to hyperventilation and therefore is suffering from a respiratory alkalosis. In an acute respiratory alkalosis, the bicarbonate typically decreases by 2 mM for each 10 mmHg decrease in P_{CO_2}; in a chronic respiratory alkalosis the bicarbonate typically decreases by 4 mM for each 10 mmHg decrease in P_{CO_2}. In this case the P_{CO_2} has decreased by 30 mmHg. Because bicarbonate has decreased by 12 mM, the diagnosis is consistent with a chronic respiratory alkalosis.

318. The answer is c. *(Boron, pp 410–411, 641. Guyton.)* Reducing alveolar ventilation will decrease the pH toward a normal value. However, in this circumstance, it is an inappropriate therapy because the high pH is keeping most of the aspirin in an ionized form in which it cannot easily cross the blood-brain barrier. When the patient was placed on a ventilator, to prevent muscle fatigue, the hyperventilation was not sustained, the aspirin crossed the blood brain barrier, and the situation became far worse.

319. The answer is d. *(Boron, pp 747–749.)* The fractional excretion is the fraction of the filtered load that is excreted. It is calculated using the formula

$$FE = \frac{\text{Amount Excreted}}{\text{Amount Filtered}} = \frac{U_{Na} \times \dot{V}}{P_{Na} \times GFR}; \text{ Since } GFR = \frac{U_{Creatinine} \times \dot{V}}{P_{Creatinine}}$$

$$FE = \frac{U_{Na} \times \dot{V}}{P_{Na} \times \dfrac{U_{Creatinine} \times \dot{V}}{P_{Creatinine}}} = \frac{U_{Na} \times P_{Creatinine}}{P_{Na} \times U_{Creatinine}} = \frac{33 \text{ mM} \times 7.5 \text{ mg/dL}}{135 \text{ mM} \times 90 \text{ mg/dL}} = 0.02$$

Fractional excretion is used to distinguish between volume depletion and acute renal failure. A fractional excretion of less than 1% is consistent with volume depletion, whereas a fractional excretion greater than 2% is consistent with acute renal failure. This patient, with a fraction excretion of 2%, was diagnosed with acute renal failure caused by excessive intake of Motrin.

320. The answer is d. *(Boron, pp 846–847.)* Net acid excretion is the amount of acid excreted each day. It is calculated using the formula

$$\text{Net Acid Excretion (NAE)} = (\text{TA} - \text{NH}_4^+ - \text{HCO}_3^-) \times \dot{V}$$

$$\text{NAE} = (24 \text{ meq/L} + 38 \text{ meq/L} - 2 \text{ meq/L}) \times 1.2 \text{ L/day} = 72 \text{ meq/L}$$

Almost all of the acid excreted is buffered by either phosphate, called titratable acid, and ammonia. The titratable acid is equal to the mM of NaOH that must be added to the urine to raise its pH back to that of plasma. Bicarbonate must be subtracted from the sum of acid excreted because each milliequivalent of excreted bicarbonate represents the addition of 1 meq of acid to the plasma.

321. The answer is c. (*Boron, pp 767–769. Guyton, pp 309–310.*) The clearance of PAH is a good estimate of renal plasma flow (RPF) because, under normal circumstances, almost all (more than 90%) of the PAH passing through the kidney is excreted.

$$C_{\text{PAH}} = \frac{U_{\text{PAH}} \times \dot{V}}{P_{\text{PAH}}} = \frac{25 \text{ mg/mL} \times 1.5 \text{ mL/min}}{6 \text{ mg/dL}} = 625 \text{ mL/min}$$

If the clearance of PAH is 90% of the actual renal blood flow, then the true renal blood flow is approximately 695 mL/min.

322. The answer is d. (*Boron, pp 766–769. Guyton, p 309.*) If a substance disappears from the circulation during its passage through the kidney, it usually indicates that it has been totally secreted into the nephron. In this case, its clearance will be equal to the RPF. If the substance is bound to plasma proteins, it can be secreted without being filtered. Even if it is entirely secreted by the kidney, its urinary concentration may be less than its plasma concentration if the urinary flow rate is very high.

323. The answer is c. (*Boron, pp 758–760. Guyton, pp 309–312.*) Because the amount of fluid excreted by the kidney is only a small fraction of the renal plasma flow, the volume of fluid in the vein is essentially equal to that in the artery. Thus, the difference between the arterial and venous concentrations is due to the loss of solute. Because the material is neither reabsorbed nor secreted, its removal from the plasma must have been by glomerular filtration. Therefore the filtered solute equals 12 mg/ml − 9 mg/ml, and the percent of the arterial concentration that is filtered (and therefore, the fraction of plasma filtered) is

$$\frac{3 \text{ mg/mL}}{12 \text{ mg/mL}} = 0.25$$

324. The answer is a. (*Boron, p 843. Guyton, p 322.*) The inflammatory process affected the ability of the posterior pituitary to secrete ADH. Therefore the patient developed diabetes insipidus, which would result in the excretion of a high volume of urine (polyuria) with a low tonicity.

325. The answer is e. (*Boron, p 641. Guyton, pp 358–363.*) The low FVC (forced vital capacity) with a normal FEV_1/FVC ratio indicates a severe restrictive lung disease resulting in hypoventilation and consequently a respiratory acidosis. Respiratory acidosis is characterized by a low arterial pH and a high arterial bicarbonate concentration. The alveolar-arterial gradient will most likely be in the normal range unless the respiratory disease leads to a V/Q abnormality. Pectus excavatum (PE) is defined as an abnormal formation of the rib cage where the breastbone caves in, resulting in a sunken chest appearance. It was responsible for the restrictive lung disease.

326. The answer is e. (*Boron, pp 852–853. Guyton, pp 353–355.*) The pH of the tubular fluid in the distal nephron can be lower than that in the proximal tubule because the tight junctions between the cells in the distal nephron are "tighter," or less leaky, than those in the proximal tubule. A H^+ ion gradient of only 10 to 1 (i.e., a minimum luminal pH of about 6.4) can be established in the proximal tubule, whereas a H^+ ion gradient of 1000 to 1 (i.e., a minimum luminal pH of 4.4) can be established in the distal nephron. Because of the tighter junctions, the distal nephron can also establish a greater sodium gradient. Even though the distal nephron can maintain a lower luminal pH, a lesser volume of H^+ ions is actually secreted than in the proximal tubule. The distal nephron, unlike the proximal tubule, does not have a true brush border, and there is no carbonic anhydrase on the luminal surface of the cells as in the proximal tubule.

327. The answer is d. (*Boron, pp 745–746. Guyton, pp 201–206.*) Renin is secreted by the juxtaglomerular cells (near the afferent arterioles) in response to decreased renal arterial pressure. It acts on angiotensinogen to form angiotensin I. Angiotensin I is then converted to angiotensin II, a highly potent pressor agent that, despite a short half-life in humans, has numerous regulatory functions, including the control of aldosterone secretion and sodium and water conservation.

328. The answer is d. (*Guyton, pp 310–311.*) Free water clearance is the amount of water excreted in excess of that required to excrete urine that is isoosmotic to plasma. A negative free water clearance indicates that the amount of water is less than that required to excrete urine that is isoosmotic to plasma. It is calculated using the formula:

$$\text{Free Water Clearance } (C_{H_2O}) = \dot{V} - C_{osmolar}$$

$$C_{osmolar} = \frac{U_{osm} \times \dot{V}}{P_{osm}}; U_{osm} = 2 \times [Na^+] + [K^+]$$

$$C_{H_2O} = \dot{V} - \frac{2 \times ([Na^+] + [K^+]) \times \dot{V}}{P_{osm}}$$

$$C_{H_2O} = 1 \text{ L/day} - \frac{2 \times (125 \text{ mM} + 25 \text{ mM}) \times 1 \text{ L/day}}{2 \times 125 \text{ mM}}$$

$$C_{H_2O} = -0.2 \text{ L/day}$$

This patient has a negative free water clearance, which means she is diluting her plasma despite her low serum sodium. The urine osmolarity is estimated from the concentration of sodium and potassium because these electrolytes determine the shift of water between intracellular and extracellular compartments. The measured osmolarity is not used because it includes urea, which has no effect on body fluid distribution. The serum hypotonicity (250mosmol/L) causes brain swelling, accounting for her signs and symptoms. The negative free water clearance is probably caused by the combination of diuretics and antidepressants, which stimulate the release of ADH.

329. The answer is e. (*Guyton, pp 360, 377.*) The rise in H^+ and fall in HCO_3^- that occurs in type I (distal) renal tubular acidosis (RTA) does not increase the anion gap because the decrease in HCO_3^- is accompanied by an increase in Cl. The failure of the distal nephron H^+ ATPase causes a reduction in net acid excretion and a reduced H^+ secretion, which causes less ammonium to be excreted in the urine. The low HCO_3^- in the glomerular filtrate reduces Na^+ reabsorption by Na-H exchanger and therefore more

Na^+ is delivered to the distal nephron. The increased Na^+ delivery results in salt wasting and a secondary hyperaldosteronism which, in turn, causes K^+ concentration to fall.

330. The answer is b. *(Boron, pp 47–748, 767–769. Guyton, p 311.)* The clearance of PAH equals the true renal plasma flow only if the kidney reabsorbs all of the filtered PAH, that is, no PAH appears in the renal vein. Because the kidney is only able to reabsorb approximately 85 to 90% of the filtered PAH, some PAH appears in the renal vein, and the PAH clearance is less than the true renal plasma flow.

331. The answer is a. *(Boron, pp 792–795. Guyton, pp 298–299.)* Glucose reabsorption employs an active transport mechanism located in the proximal tubule. The same mechanism also transports fructose, galactose, and xylose. Essentially all filtered glucose is reabsorbed, inasmuch as the transport maximum (T_{max}) for glucose (320 mg/min) is not exceeded in normal persons. In diabetes mellitus, hyperglycemia results in a tubular filtration load that exceeds the T_{max}, and glycosuria ensues.

332. The answer is c. *(Boron, pp 739–745. Guyton, pp 300–305.)* The major structural differences between epithelial cells of the proximal and distal tubules account for the fact that 65% of glomerular filtrate is reabsorbed in the proximal tubule and that the proximal tubule is more permeable to water. The proximal tubule has an extensive brush border composed of numerous microvilli, which markedly increase the surface area for reabsorption, and the tubule also has an extensive network of intracellular channels. The distal tubule has many more tight junctions between cells, which makes it less permeable to water. No significant difference in basement membrane thickness is observed between the proximal and distal tubules. Cells of the distal tubule lying adjacent to the afferent arteriole form the juxtaglomerular apparatus.

333. The answer is e. *(Boron, pp 284–286, 373, 760–763.)* Approximately two-thirds of the 40 to 150 mg of protein excreted per day by the kidney is derived from plasma proteins. The remainder is derived from the tubular secretion of a mucoprotein, the Tamm-Horsfall protein, that is present in tubular casts appearing in urinary sediment. Not all plasma proteins are filtered equally because glomerular permeability is related to molecular size and charge. The larger and negatively charged proteins are poorly filtered. Most of the filtered protein is reabsorbed in the proximal tubule unless the filtered load exceeds the tubular capacity. Such overload would occur following damage to the glomerular basement membrane and breakdown of normal barriers, or following an increase in the plasma concentration of a small protein, such as myoglobin. Protein excretion is also increased by sympathetic stimulation, such as that occurring during exercise. In this situation, renal vasoconstriction reduces the glomerular filtration rate, which, by increasing the transit time of glomerular filtrate, favors diffusion of proteins across the basement membrane.

334. The answer is a. (*Boron, pp 762–765. Guyton, pp 286–288.*) The renal artery pressure and the resistance of the renal vascular bed determine renal blood flow. Decreasing the resistance of either the afferent or efferent arterioles could increase RBF. Alternatively, if the resistance of one of these vessels decreased more than the resistance of the other one increased, RBF would also increase. Glomerular filtration rate will increase if glomerular capillary pressure increases. This can occur if the afferent arteriolar resistance decreases or if the efferent arteriolar resistance increases.

335. The answer is d. (*Boron, pp 79–81. Guyton, pp 269–273.*) Drinking water after losing a significant volume of water as sweat decreases the osmolarity of the extracellular fluid. The decrease occurs because the salt lost from the extracellular fluid in sweat is not replaced by the ingested water. When the extracellular osmolarity is decreased, water flows from the extracellular to the intracellular body compartment, causing intracellular volume to increase. The patient's symptoms are caused by swelling of the brain.

336. The answer is e. (*Boron, pp 854–857. Guyton, pp 356–357.*) Ammonia (NH_3) is produced from amino acids in the cells of the renal tubules (mainly the proximal tubules), and its rate of production increases during acidosis. This is important in acidosis because it increases the total amount of H^+ ion that can be excreted in a given volume of urine. The NH_3 freely diffuses into the tubular lumen, and because of the high pK_a (9.2) of the reaction, essentially all of it combines with H^+ to form NH_4^+. This maintains the driving force for more NH_3 to passively diffuse into the lumen. The NH_4^+ that is formed gets "trapped" in the tubules and excreted because the tubules are impermeable to this cation.

337. The answer is d. *(Boron, pp 822–827. Guyton, pp 338–342.)* The amount of potassium excreted is controlled by the amount of potassium secreted by the distal tubule. Potassium secretion is a passive process that depends on the electrochemical gradient between the distal tubular cells and the tubular lumen and the permeability of the luminal cells to potassium. By inhibiting Na^+ reabsorption, the intraluminal potential becomes less negative and K^+ secretion is reduced. K^+-sparing diuretics such as amiloride act in this fashion. Aldosterone increases the intracellular potassium concentration by augmenting the activity of the Na-K pump and increasing the potassium permeability of the luminal membrane. Increasing dietary intake increases the plasma potassium concentration, which in turn stimulates aldosterone production. Increasing the rate of distal tubular flow increases the rate of K^+ secretion. The high flow maintains a low tubular K^+ concentration and therefore increases the electrochemical gradient for K^+ secretion.

338. The answer is a. *(Boron, pp 640–641, 729–730. Guyton, pp 351–352.)* Increasing arterial pH stimulates both the central and peripheral chemoreceptors. The increased arterial hydrogen ion concentration increases H^+ secretion by the distal tubule, lowering the pH of the urine and increasing the excretion of NH_4^+ excretion. The excretion of H^+ is accompanied by the generation of new bicarbonate, causing the plasma HCO_3^- to increase.

339. The answer is b. *(Boron, pp 830–831. Guyton, pp 300–302.)* Sodium is isosmotically reabsorbed from the proximal tubule; that is, when sodium is reabsorbed, water flows out of the proximal tubule to maintain a constant osmolarity. Thus, the concentration of sodium does not normally change as the filtrate flows through the proximal tubule. Because creatinine cannot be reabsorbed from the tubule, its concentration rises as water is reabsorbed. The concentration of glucose, bicarbonate, and phosphate are all less at the end of the proximal tubule than at the beginning.

340. The answer is c. *(Boron, pp 830–831, 839–841. Guyton, pp 314–315.)* When a person is dehydrated, ADH secretion increases. In the presence of ADH, the cortical and medullary collecting tubules become permeable to water, and the filtrate within these portions of the nephron reaches osmotic equilibrium with the interstitial fluid surrounding them. The ascending limb of the loop of Henle is not affected by ADH and so remains impermeable to water. As sodium and other electrolytes are reabsorbed from the ascending limb, its filtrate becomes hypotonic. The glomerular filtrate and proximal tubular fluid remain isotonic to plasma, which in the case of dehydration is higher than normal.

341. The answer is a. *(Boron, pp 774–781. Guyton, pp 302–303.)* Na$^+$ and Cl$^-$ are reabsorbed from the distal convoluted tubule by an electrically neutral carrier. The thick ascending limb of Henle's loop employs a carrier that binds one sodium, one potassium, and two chloride ions. It is also electrically neutral. Na$^+$ diffusion through channels on the apical surface of principal cells of the cortical and medullary collecting ducts is electrogenic.

342. The answer is b. *(Boron, pp 3–54, 1084. Guyton, pp 362–363.)* In diabetic ketoacidosis, there is an increased production of acetoacetic and β-hydroxybutyric acids, which leads to an increase in plasma concentration of hydrogen ion. These fixed acids are buffered by all body buffers but mainly by bicarbonate. The concentration of plasma HCO_3^- is therefore below normal. The consumption of bicarbonate and the addition of the anions of the fixed acids to the plasma cause an elevation of the anion gap. The anion gap is equal to plasma [Na$^+$] − (plasma [HCO_3^-] + plasma [Cl$^-$]) and is normally about 12 to 15 meq/L. The acidosis would stimulate the carotid body chemoreceptors (and eventually the central chemoreceptors) to cause an increase in ventilation, which decreases arterial PCO_2. Although blood volume is not affected by metabolic acidosis, the osmotic diuresis that accompanies untreated diabetes may lead to a loss of blood volume.

343. The answer is e. *(Boron, pp 762–765.)* Renal plasma flow, filtration fraction, the oncotic pressure, and the filtration rate all increase when the afferent arteriolar resistance is decreased. The renal blood flow increases because total renal resistance is less. Decreasing renal resistance also increases the glomerular capillary pressure, which results in an increase in filtration fraction. Because more fluid is filtered out of the glomerular capillaries and no plasma protein is removed, the oncotic pressure rises. The glomerular filtration rate (GFR) is proportional to the glomerular capillary pressure and the renal plasma flow (RPF). Because both of these increase, so does the GFR.

344. The answer is c. (*Boron, pp 783–786.*) When water is filtered across the glomerulus, the protein concentration (the oncotic pressure) within the capillaries increases, which in turn increases the efficiency by which water reabsorbed from the proximal tubule is returned to the circulatory system. If GFR increases, it results in a larger increase in oncotic pressure. This in turn increases the amount of water reabsorbed from the proximal tubule.

345. The answer is e. (*Boron, pp 745–746. Guyton, pp 200–202, 290–292.*) Juxtaglomerular (JG) cells are sensitive to changes in afferent arterial intraluminal pressure. Increased pressure within the afferent arteriole leads to a decrease in renin release, whereas decreased pressure tends to increase renin release. Angiotensin appears to inhibit renin release by initiating the flow of calcium into the JG cells. Renin release is increased in response to increased activity in the sympathetic neurons innervating the kidney. Prostaglandins, particularly PGI_2 and PGE_2, stimulate renin release. Stimulation of the macula densa leads to an increase in renin release, and although the mechanism is not fully understood, it appears that increased delivery of NaCl to the distal nephron is responsible for stimulating the macula densa. Aldosterone does not appear to have any direct effect on renin release.

346. The answer is d. (*Boron, pp 46, 772. Guyton, pp 373–376.*) Most urea is synthesized in the liver. Its excretion is dependent on its concentration in plasma and the glomerular filtration rate (GFR) in the kidney. Approximately 50 to 60% of filtered plasma urea is passively reabsorbed in the proximal tubule at normal GFR. In renal insufficiency, in which GFR is decreased, less urea is filtered and therefore less urea is excreted. The decreased excretion of urea results in an increase in its plasma concentration.

347. The answer is b. (*Boron, pp 1058–1059.*) Aldosterone binds to an intracellular receptor that causes an increased synthesis of a variety of proteins, including K^+ and Na^+ ion channels and Na^+-K^+-ATPase, which together act to increase Na^+ reabsorption and K^+ secretion by the tubular cells of the distal nephron. H^+ secretion is also enhanced by aldosterone. Aldosterone secretion is stimulated by a decrease in blood volume (through the renin-angiotensin system) and by increased plasma K^+ concentrations.

High blood pressure, if it has any effect on aldosterone, will cause a decrease in its secretion.

348. The answer is a. (*Boron, pp 840–844, 870–871.*) The principal physiologic action of ADH is to increase water retention by the kidney. The hormone acts on the distal nephron to increase its permeability so that water more readily enters the hypertonic interstitium of the renal pyramids. Thus, the concentration of solutes in the urine is increased. ADH increases Na^+ reabsorption so that the actual amount of Na^+ excreted is decreased. It also acts as a vasoconstrictor; hence, it is called arginine vasopressin (AVP). ADH has no effect on glomerular filtration rate, and because it increases water reabsorption, it would decrease urine formation.

349. The answer is d. (*Boron, pp 648–649, 1084.*) The normal compensation for metabolic acidosis is hyperventilation and decreased P_{CO_2}. This patient exhibited hypoventilation because of muscle weakness. The muscle weakness was secondary to the high plasma potassium concentration. Hyperkalemia is frequently observed in patients with uncontrolled diabetic ketoacidosis. The hyperosmotic extracellular fluid draws water out of cells. K^+ follows the water by solvent drag. Additionally, the lack of insulin decreases the ability of K^+ to enter cells. The high anion gap is produced by the ketoacids. Bicarbonate levels are reduced by the metabolic acidosis.

350. The answer is d. (*Boron, pp 830–836. Guyton, pp 319–320.*) Concentrated urine is produced by the reabsorption of water from the medullary collecting ducts down an osmotic gradient that is created by the reabsorption of sodium from the loop of Henle. If the Na^+-K^+ pump activity in the loop of Henle is increased, the osmotic gradient, and the ability to excrete concentrated urine, is increased. Water reabsorption will be reduced if the permeability of the collecting duct principal cells is reduced. Also, concentrated urine will be more difficult to produce if an increase in glomerular capillary increases the filtered load of Na^+ or if the reabsorption of Na^+ is decreased in the proximal tubule.

351. The answer is d. (*Boron, pp 752–754. Guyton, pp 364–365.*) This patient developed acute renal failure due to uretal obstruction. Uretal obstruction is indicated by the swelling of the kidneys. The uretal obstruction raises the hydrostatic pressure within Bowman's space, which reduces glomerular filtration. The decrease in GFR (postrenal renal failure) produces the increases creatinine. The normal blood pressure rules out sympathetic discharge, coarctation of the renal artery, and hypovolemia as causes of her renal failure. Hyperproteinemia, although possibly a cause of renal failure, would not produce an enlarged kidney.

352. The answer is a. *(Boron, pp 823–824, 859. Guyton, pp 360, 873.)* Aldosterone promotes the loss of both H^+ and K^+, producing metabolic alkalosis and hypokalemia. Persistent diarrhea will cause the loss of bicarbonate from the body, resulting in metabolic acidosis. Renal failure is often accompanied by metabolic acidosis because of the inability to excrete H^+. Diabetes also causes metabolic acidosis because of the accumulation of keto acids. Hyperventilation results in a respiratory alkalosis, which is compensated for by a decreased bicarbonate concentration.

353. The answer is b. *(Boron, p 844.)* The increased secretion of antidiuretic hormone (ADH) increases the permeability of the distal nephron to water and therefore increases the reabsorption of water from the kidney. The excessive reabsorption of water dilutes the extracellular fluid, producing a decrease in plasma sodium, osmolarity, and oncotic pressure. The decreased extracellular osmolarity causes water to flow from the extracellular fluid compartment into the intracellular fluid compartment, increasing intracellular volume. Because more water is being reabsorbed, less is excreted and urinary flow is decreased.

354. The answer is c. *(Boron, pp 743–744, 817–822, 849–851.)* The distal nephron has a negative luminal potential because it is poorly permeable to negatively charged ions. Therefore, when Na^+ is reabsorbed, negatively charged ions, primarily Cl^-, lag behind, producing a negative intraluminal potential. Although a similar situation occurs in the proximal tubule, the proximal tubule has a higher permeability to Cl^- and, therefore, does not develop as large a negative intraluminal potential. The distal nephron is less permeable to hydrogen than the proximal tubule. Aldosterone increases Na^+ reabsorption from the distal nephron but has no effect on the proximal tubule. K^+ is reabsorbed from the proximal tubule and secreted by the distal nephron. Although the amount of H^+ excreted each day is determined by the amount of H^+ secreted into the distal nephron, the proximal tubule secretes much more H^+ than the distal nephron. However, almost all of the H^+ secreted in the proximal tubule is reabsorbed in association with the reabsorption of HCO_3^-.

355. The answer is c. (*Boron, pp 745–746, 769–761.*) The macula densa senses the chloride concentration of the fluid flowing from the ascending limb of Henle's loop into the distal convoluted tubule. An increase in NaCl concentration occurs when the amount of fluid flowing through the ascending limb increases because there is less time available for the reabsorption of NaCl. The resulting increase in Cl^- concentration results in the release of adenosine (and/or ATP) from the macula densa. Adenosine constricts the afferent arteriole, resulting in a decrease in filtration and a return of the flow rate within the nephron toward normal. This response is referred to as tubuloglomerular feedback. If the NaCl concentration decreases, for example, when circulating blood volume decreases, the decreased Cl^- concentration results in the release of renin from granular cells of the juxtaglomerular apparatus.

356. The answer is a. (*Boron, p 859. Guyton, pp 360–361, 872–874.*) Hypoaldosteronism (Addison's disease) results in a decrease in H^+ secretion, which leads to the production of a metabolic acidosis. Hyperventilation produces a respiratory acidosis, which is compensated for by an increase in bicarbonate reabsorption, yielding a metabolic alkalosis. Hypokalemia causes an increase in K^+ reabsorption and an increase in H^+ secretion, resulting in a metabolic alkalosis. Hypovolemia results in an increase in aldosterone secretion, which can lead to an increase in H^+ secretion and a metabolic alkalosis.

357. The answer is e. (*Boron, pp 1059–1061. Guyton, pp 340–341.*) The synthesis and secretion of aldosterone are dependent primarily on the renin-angiotensin system. Increased potassium concentration directly stimulates aldosterone secretion. Increased circulating blood volume leads to a decrease in renin secretion and therefore a decrease in aldosterone secretion. The role of adrenocorticotropic hormone (ACTH) in aldosterone synthesis and secretion is negligible.

358. The answer is c. (*Boron, pp 771–772. Guyton, pp 332–333.*) The rate of fluid volume excretion is influenced by the glomerular filtration rate

(GFR) and the rate of tubular reabsorption. Increased renal arterial pressure increases urinary volume by increasing GFR, whereas sympathetic stimulation, by causing vasoconstriction, decreases both GFR and urinary volume. An increase in the filtered load of an osmotically active solute that is not reabsorbed, such as the nonmetabolized carbohydrate mannitol, or that is filtered in excess of the tubular capacity, such as glucose in diabetes mellitus, will decrease water resorption in parallel, and an osmotic diuresis will ensue. In diabetes insipidus, ADH secretion is markedly reduced or absent, and water passes through the relatively impermeable collecting ducts without being reabsorbed.

359. The answer is c. (*Boron, pp 642–644.*) A large amount of volatile acid (carbon dioxide) is produced by aerobic metabolism. The lungs excrete almost all of the CO_2 as it is formed. Nonbicarbonate buffers, primarily hemoglobin, buffer any CO_2 that accumulates in the blood. Phosphate, lactate, and plasma proteins are also nonbicarbonate buffers, but they buffer only a small portion of the volatile acid dissolving in the blood.

360. The answer is d. (*Boron, pp 823–824, 859–860. Guyton, pp 367–368.*) Diuretics produce an increase in water excretion primarily by blocking Na^+ reabsorption. If Na^+ reabsorption is blocked in the proximal portions of the nephron, then the amount of Na^+ in the filtrate flowing through the distal nephron increases. The increased Na^+ load in the distal nephron results in an increased Na^+ reabsorption and, as a result, an increased K^+ secretion. If Na^+ reabsorption in the distal nephron is blocked, then a diuresis can be produced without an excess loss of K^+. These diuretics, some of which block the aldosterone receptor, others of which block the Na channels on the apical surface of the distal nephron tubular cells, are called potassium-sparing diuretics.

361. The answer is a. (*Boron, pp 782, 831–833. Guyton, pp 367–368.*) The increase in blood glucose concentration will result in a filtered load of glucose in excess of what the proximal tubule is able to absorb. As a result, glucose will remain in the filtrate, where it will act as an osmotic diuretic increasing urinary flow. The excess blood glucose will cause water to shift from the intracellular compartment to the extracellular compartment, causing a decrease in intracellular volume and, by dilution, a decrease in plasma sodium concentration. The accompanying increase in ketoacid production will result in a metabolic acidosis (low pH) and a compensatory increase in alveolar ventilation, lowering alveolar P_{CO_2}.

362. The answer is c. (*Boron, pp 857–858. Guyton, pp 358–360.*) Persistent diarrhea will result in a metabolic acidosis, due to the loss of the bicarbonate-rich secretions from the pancreas and gallbladder. The ensuing metabolic acidosis will decrease the plasma concentration of HCO_3^-, decreasing the amount of bicarbonate that is filtered into the proximal tubule. At the same time, the metabolic acidosis will increase ammonia production by the proximal tubule as well as H^+ secretion and production of new bicarbonate by the distal nephron. Because the metabolic acidosis is produced by the loss of bicarbonate, the anion gap will remain within normal limits.

363. The answer is e. (*Boron, pp 42–844. Guyton, p 319.*) ADH increases the permeability of the distal nephron to urea as well as to water. The increased urea permeability increases the urea concentration and osmolarity of the interstitial fluid surrounding the loop of Henle and the distal nephron. The high interstitial urea concentration helps to increase the osmolarity of the fluid within the descending limb of the loop of Henle, the reabsorption of Na^+ from the ascending limb of the loop of Henle, and the reabsorption of water from the distal nephron.

364. The answer is c. (*Boron, pp 763–765, 784–785. Guyton, pp 284–287.*) The filtration fraction is directly proportional to the glomerular capillary pressure. Increasing the resistance of the efferent arteriole increases the glomerular capillary pressure and, therefore, the filtration fraction. Increasing renal blood flow will not have any direct effect on the filtration fraction but may cause the filtration fraction to decrease if the excess flow rate through the glomerulus limits the amount of filtration that can occur. Increasing the afferent arteriolar resistance will decrease glomerular capillary pressure and, therefore, the filtration fraction. Increasing the plasma oncotic pressure or the hydrostatic pressure within Bowman's capsule will decrease the filtration fraction because both of these Starling forces oppose filtration.

365. The answer is a. (*Boron, pp 856–860.*) Under normal circumstances, the kidney reabsorbs enough bicarbonate to keep the plasma concentration at 24 meq/L and excretes the rest. Therefore, bicarbonate concentrations cannot be increased very much by infusing HCO_3^-. An increase in plasma bicarbonate concentration requires a deficit in the normal excretory function or, what amounts to the same thing, an increase in bicarbonate reabsorptive capacity. Volume depletion activates the renin-angiotensin-aldosterone system. Angiotensin II increases bicarbonate reabsorption in the proximal tubule by increasing Na/H exchange, and aldosterone increases distal bicarbonate reabsorption by promoting H^+ secretion. Renal failure, hypoxemia, and diarrhea all produce metabolic acidosis accompanied by a decreased plasma bicarbonate concentration.

366. The answer is d. *(Boron, pp 769–772.)* Blood flow through the kidney is controlled by a myriad of humoral agents. Adenosine acts via A_2 receptors to increase afferent arteriolar resistance and thereby decrease renal blood flow. Nitric oxide dilates the afferent arteriole and constricts the efferent arteriole, producing a rise in glomerular capillary pressure (and glomerular filtration) without having much of an effect on renal blood flow. Prostaglandins, bradykinin, and dopamine all increase renal blood flow. Cyclooxygenase inhibitors, such as aspirin, that decrease prostaglandin synthesis may impair renal blood flow sufficiently to exacerbate the effects of renal failure.

367. The answer is a. *(Boron, p 853. Guyton, pp 367–369.)* Carbonic anhydrase is the enzyme that catalyzes the formation of CO_2 and H_2O from HCO_3^- and H^+. In the proximal tubule, the efficient reabsorption of bicarbonate requires the presence of carbonic anhydrase. Carbonic anhydrase inhibitors prevent the formation of CO_2 and therefore block the reabsorption of bicarbonate (and Na^+), resulting in a diuresis. Because almost all of the filtered bicarbonate is reabsorbed in the proximal tubule, inhibiting carbonic anhydrase has little effect on bicarbonate reabsorption from other segments of the nephron.

368. The answer is b. *(Boron, pp 814–816.)* The movement of K^+ into cells is facilitated by the presence of insulin and epinephrine. During exercise, epinephrine hastens the movement of K^+ into muscle cells, preventing the accumulation of K^+ in the extracellular space around active muscle cells. In cases of life-threatening hyperkalemia, insulin is often injected (along with glucose) to reduce K^+ concentration.

369. The answer is b. (*Boron, pp 644–650. Guyton, pp 357–360.*) The analysis of blood gases can suggest the presence of an acid-base disturbance, but an exact diagnosis requires knowledge of the complete clinical condition. A metabolic acidosis is characterized by a lower than normal pH (acidemia) accompanied by a decrease in bicarbonate and a decrease in arterial P_{CO_2}. The lower than normal bicarbonate concentration (less than 24 meq/L) is produced by the buffering of fixed acids by bicarbonate, and the lower than normal arterial P_{CO_2} (less than 40 mmHg) is produced by respiratory compensation for the acidemia. If the acidemia is accompanied by a higher than normal arterial P_{CO_2} and a higher than normal bicarbonate concentration, respiratory acidosis is the most likely cause.

370. The answer is a. (*Boron, pp 822–827. Guyton, pp 336–342.*) Hyperkalemia can be caused by increased consumption or decreased excretion. Pathophysiologically, chronic hyperkalemia is almost always due to decreased excretion. Decreased excretion most commonly occurs in renal failure of volume depletion. The amount of potassium excreted each day depends primarily on the amount of potassium secreted by the distal nephron. Secretion will decrease in renal failure because there are less functional nephrons (although the functioning nephrons secrete a greater amount of potassium). Hypokalemia can result from an increase in excretion, as may occur when diuretics are administered. Hypokalemia can also result from sequestration of extracellular potassium into cells, as may occur in metabolic alkalosis, elevated epinephrine concentration, or administration of insulin.

371. The answer is a. (*Boron, pp 646–650. Guyton, pp 359–363, 496–498.*) When a person ascends to high altitudes, the low oxygen produces hypoxemia, which causes a respiratory alkalosis (low P_{CO_2}). Bicarbonate concentrations fall to compensate for the metabolic alkalosis. The low oxygen may produce a metabolic (lactic) acidosis, further lowering the bicarbonate concentration. The only set of blood gases with low P_{CO_2} and low bicarbonate is located at point **A** on the graph.

372. The answer is d. (*Boron, pp 779–781. Guyton, pp 300–302.*) The proximal tubule reabsorbs approximately two-thirds of the filtered water and two-thirds of the filtered Na^+, Cl^-, and K^+. Therefore, the concentration of these substances is the same at the beginning and end of the proximal tubule. Because creatinine is not reabsorbed, its concentration increases from the proximal to distal ends of the proximal tubule. Phosphate, however, is almost completely reabsorbed in the proximal tubule, so its concentration decreases along the length of the tubule.

373. The answer is d. *(Boron, pp 777–778, 783–786. Guyton, pp 300–302.)* About two-thirds of the filtered load of sodium is reabsorbed by the proximal tubule. This percentage is maintained when there are spontaneous changes in the filtered load by a process called glomerular tubular balance. However, the percentage of reabsorption can be changed when necessary to maintain homeostasis. For example, the production of angiotensin II during volume depletion can result in the reabsorption of as much as 75% of the filtered load of Na^+.

374. The answer is e. *(Boron, pp 787–788.)* Atrial natriuretic peptide (ANP) increases Na^+ excretion by decreasing the amount of Na^+ reabsorbed from the inner medullary collecting duct by decreasing the permeability of the apical membrane of the collecting duct epithelial cells. Less Na^+ is able to enter the epithelial cells and therefore, less Na is reabsorbed. ANP also increases Na^+ excretion by increasing the filtered load of Na^+.

375. The answer is e. *(Boron, pp 829–830. Guyton, pp 321–322.)* Free water clearance is the amount of water excreted in excess of that required to make the urine isotonic to plasma. It is calculated using the formula: $C_{H_2O} = \dot{V} - C_{osm}$. Free water clearance is positive when the urine is dilute (more than a sufficient amount of water is excreted), and free water clearance is negative when the urine is concentrated (not enough water is excreted to make the urine isotonic to plasma). An increase in free water clearance can lead to hypernatremia; a decrease in free water clearance can lead to hyponatremia. In diabetes insipidus, very little water is reabsorbed in the distal nephron, and, therefore, the free water clearance is very high. In heart failure or renal failure, very little free water can be generated even if the urine is dilute because the glomerular filtration rate is decreased. With diuretic therapy, Na^+ excretion is increased. Therefore, the increased water excretion is accompanied by an increased Na^+ excretion and the amount of free water generated is limited. Although the water loss is proportionally greater than the solute loss in diabetes mellitus, the amount of water excreted is much less and the solute concentration significantly higher than in diabetes insipidus, so the free water clearance is much less in diabetes mellitus than in diabetes insipidus.

376. The answer is b. (*Boron, pp 804–807. Guyton, pp 900–901, 907–910.*) Between 85 and 90% of the filtered phosphate is reabsorbed in the proximal tubule by a sodium-dependent secondary active transport system. The transporter is electrically neutral, requiring 2 Na^+ molecules for every HPO_4^{2-} molecule that it transports. The transporter is inhibited by parathyroid hormone (PTH). The decreased reabsorption of phosphate results in an increased clearance from the plasma. PTH is released from the parathyroid gland in response to lowered plasma Ca^{2+} concentrations. In addition to inhibiting the reabsorption of phosphate from the proximal tubule, PTH increases the reabsorption of Ca^{2+} from the loop of Henle.

377. The answer is a. (*Boron, p 844.*) Vasopressin (AVP or ADH) increases water reabsorption from the cortical and medullary collecting ducts in the kidney. ADH is normally released in response to a rise in plasma Na^+ concentration, and therefore the increased water reabsorption appropriately restores extracellular osmolarity toward normal. When excess ADH is excreted, the water reabsorption dilutes the extracellular fluid, producing hyponatremia. This condition is called the syndrome of inappropriate ADH secretion (SIADH) and can be life-threatening.

378. The answer is b. (*Boron, pp 823–827.*) Potassium is secreted from the principle cells lining the cortical and medullary collecting ducts. Secretion is passive and is increased by increasing the electrochemical gradient driving the diffusion through the potassium channels on the apical surface of the principle cells. Increasing Na^+ concentration within the distal nephron increases Na^+ reabsorption, which, in turn, increases the negativity of the luminal electrical potential. The increased negativity drives K^+ into the lumen at a greater rate. Decreasing the distal flow rate, which occurs when circulating blood volume or renal blood decreases or when sympathetic nerve activity to the renal vessels increases, will allow the K^+ concentration within the distal nephron to increase. The increase in K^+ concentration decreases the driving force for K^+ diffusion and, therefore, decreases K^+ secretion.

379. The answer is d. *(Boron, pp 866–867.)* The juxtaglomerular apparatus (JGA) is responsible for releasing renin when the effective circulating blood volume is decreased. The JGA releases renin when the Cl^- concentration in the luminal fluid bathing the macula densa is decreased. The decrease in Cl^- (and Na^+) concentration occurs when the flow rate within the nephron decreases and ample time is available for the loop of Henle to remove NaCl from the lumen. Adenosine is released from the macula densa cells when the luminal Cl^- concentration increases in response to an increase in luminal flow rate. Adenosine decreases flow rate by constricting the afferent arteriole and, therefore, the blood flow through the glomerular capillary.

380–382. The answers are 380-e, 381-d, 382-e. *(Boron, pp 786–789, 807–810. Guyton, pp 308–309, 313–315.)* The ascending limb of Henle's loop dilutes the fluid within the nephron by reabsorbing Na^+ without water. In the absence of ADH, the reabsorption of Na^+ without water continues along the collecting duct, making the Na^+ concentration lower and lower. In the presence of ADH, water is reabsorbed from the collecting duct making the luminal fluid isotonic in the cortical collecting duct and hypertonic in the medullary collecting duct.

Parathyroid hormone (PTH) increases Ca^{2+} reabsorption from the thick ascending limb and the distal convoluted tubule. Although most of the filtered Ca^{2+} is reabsorbed in the proximal tubule, the regulation of Ca^{2+} excretion occurs in the thick ascending limb and the distal convoluted tubule. PTH regulates the reabsorption of HPO_4^{2-} in the proximal tubule.

Aldosterone increases the reabsorption of Na^+ from the Principal cells within the cortical and medullary collecting ducts. Aldosterone increases Na^+ reabsorption by increasing the luminal permeability to Na^+ on the apical surface and the activity of the Na-K pump on the basal lateral surface of the Principal cells. Aldosterone also increases the secretion of K^+ and H^+ from the collecting ducts.

383. The answer is d. *(Boron, pp 769–760. Guyton, pp 371–376.)* The excretion of creatinine, which is neither reabsorbed nor secreted in any significant amount, is dependent on filtration, which is in turn dependent on renal plasma flow. The decrease in renal plasma flow that accompanies chronic renal failure results in a decrease in creatinine excretion and an increase in plasma creatinine concentration. The increase in plasma creatinine concentration is used to assess the percentage of nonfunctioning nephrons in renal failure. Interestingly, the remaining nephrons adapt to renal failure. To maintain Na^+ balance, less Na^+ is reabsorbed, so the fractional excretion (the fraction of filtered Na^+ that is excreted) goes up. Although the remaining nephrons are able to excrete a larger than normal amount of H^+, secretion cannot fully compensate for the reduced number of nephrons because there is a limit to the amount of NH_4^+ that can be synthesized by the proximal tubules. Therefore, despite the overall increase in net acid excretion, H^+ accumulation leads to a metabolic acidosis. Even creatinine secretion can be increased so the plasma creatinine concentration does not increase proportionally to the amount of renal damage. The anion gap increases because of the reduced excretion of phosphate and other anions that are included in the anion gap. Free water clearance decreases because there is decreased filtration. Therefore, to prevent overhydration in patients with renal failure, water intake must be limited.

384. The answer is c. (*Boron, pp 77–80. Guyton, pp 264–266.*) Sixty percent of the body mass is water. Of this water, one-third (20% of body mass) is extracellular and two-thirds (40% of body mass) is intracellular. The extracellular water is further divided into interstitial water (three-quarters of extracellular fluid, or 15% of body mass) and plasma water (one-fourth of extracellular fluid, or 5% of body mass). The percentage of water in the body is a function of body fat. The greater the percentage of body fat, the lower the percentage of body water. Seventy-three percent of the lean body mass (mass excluding fat) is water. The distribution of extracellular and intracellular water is a function of the extracellular osmolarity. If the osmolarity of the extracellular fluid is above normal, the proportion of water in the extracellular fluid, in comparison to that in the intracellular water, increases; hypotonicity of the extracellular water decreases the proportion of water in the extracellular fluid.

385. The answer is c. (*Boron, p 746. Guyton, pp 375–376, 385–386.*) The kidney produces a number of important hormones including vitamin D and erythropoietin. Erythropoietin is necessary for the normal production of red blood cells. The anemia associated with renal failure results from the decrease in the synthesis of erythropoietin. Often, the first clinical sign of renal failure is the fatigue produced by anemia.

386. The answer is e. *(Boron, pp 641, 648–649. Guyton, pp 360–363.)* The patient's condition is caused by a decrease in the serum concentration of ionized calcium (Ca^{2+}), which increases nerve and muscle excitability, leading to spontaneous axonal discharges and muscle contractions. Decreased Ca^{2+} concentration can result from a respiratory alkalosis because the H^+ that dissociates from plasma proteins in the presence of a high pH is replaced by Ca^{2+}. Although both a P_aCO_2 of 30 mmHg and a P_aCO_2 of 15 mmHg are consistent with respiratory alkalosis, only the combination of a P_aCO_2 of 20 mmHg and a HCO_3^- of 20 mM, produces an alkaline pH (7.6). The combination of a P_aCO_2 of 30 mmHg and a HCO_3^- of 15 mM is caused by a metabolic acidosis.

Endocrine Physiology

Questions

DIRECTIONS: Each question below contains five suggested responses. Select the **one best** response to each question.

387. The supraoptic nucleus of the hypothalamus is believed to control secretion of which of the following hormones?

a. Antidiuretic hormone (arginine vasopressin)
b. Oxytocin
c. Growth hormone
d. Adrenocorticotropic hormone
e. Follicle-stimulating hormone (FSH)

388. Parathyroid hormone (PTH) is accurately described by which of the following statements?

a. It is secreted in response to an increase in plasma Ca^{2+} concentration
b. It acts directly on bone cells to increase Ca^{2+} deposition
c. It acts directly on intestinal cells to increase Ca^{2+} absorption
d. It causes a decrease in cAMP concentration within renal proximal tubular cells
e. It is essential for life

389. Which of the following statements about spermatogenesis is correct?

a. Production and release of spermatozoa is cyclical
b. Sertoli cells are required for mitotic and meiotic activity of germ cells
c. Spermatogenesis requires continuous release of gonadotropin-releasing hormone (GRH)
d. Leydig cell secretion of testosterone requires follicle-stimulating hormone (FSH)
e. Luteinizing hormone (LH) acts directly on Sertoli cells to promote cell division

390. The secretion of growth hormone is increased by which of the following?

a. Hyperglycemia
b. Exercise
c. Somatostatin
d. Hypothermia
e. Free fatty acid

391. Which of the following is the source of estrogen and progesterone during the last seven months of pregnancy?

a. Ovary
b. Placenta
c. Corpus luteum
d. Anterior pituitary
e. Posterior pituitary

392. Which of the following is the source of estrogen and progesterone during the first two months of pregnancy?

a. Ovary
b. Placenta
c. Corpus luteum
d. Anterior pituitary
e. Posterior pituitary

393. Which one of the following hormones is secreted by the posterior pituitary gland?

a. Adrenocorticotropic hormone (ACTH)
b. Oxytocin
c. Thyroid-stimulating hormone (TSH)
d. Growth hormone (GH)
e. Prolactin

394. Which of the following statements about prolactin is correct?

a. Prolactin initiates ovulation
b. Prolactin causes milk ejection during suckling
c. Prolactin inhibits the growth of breast tissue
d. Prolactin secretion is tonically inhibited by the hypothalamus
e. Prolactin secretion is increased by dopamine

395. Which of the following is the principal steroid secreted by the fetal adrenal cortex?

a. Cortisol
b. Corticosterone
c. Dehydroepiandrosterone
d. Progesterone
e. Pregnenolone

396. The effect of insulin on glucose transport is to

a. Permit transport against a concentration gradient
b. Enhance transport into adipocytes
c. Enhance transport across the tubular epithelium of the kidney
d. Enhance transport into the brain
e. Enhance transport through the intestinal mucosa

397. The graph below demonstrates diurnal variation in the plasma level of which of the following hormones?

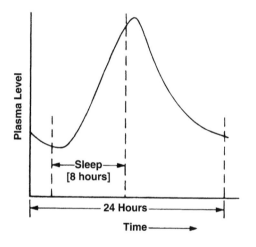

a. Thyroxine
b. Insulin
c. Parathyroid hormone
d. Cortisol
e. Estrogen

398. In the graph below showing plasma hormone levels as a function of time, ovulation takes place at which of the lettered points on the time axis?

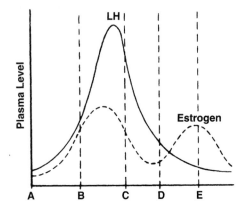

a. A
b. B
c. C
d. D
e. E

399. Iodides are stored in the thyroid follicles mainly in the form of

a. Thyroxine
b. Thyroglobulin
c. Monoiodotyrosine
d. Diiodotyrosine
e. 3,5,3'-triiodothyronine

400. The normal pattern of progesterone secretion during the menstrual cycle is exhibited by which of the following curves?

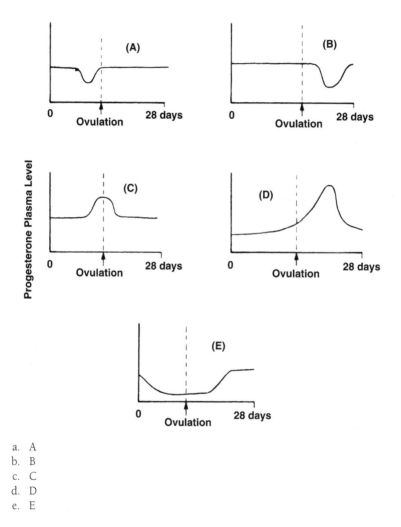

a. A
b. B
c. C
d. D
e. E

401. Almost all of the active thyroid hormone entering the circulation is in the form of

a. Triiodothyronine
b. Thyroxine
c. Thyroglobulin
d. Thyrotropin
e. Long-acting thyroid stimulator (LATS)

402. Physiologically active thyroxine exists in which of the following forms?

a. Bound to albumin
b. Bound to prealbumin
c. Bound to globulin
d. As a glucuronide
e. Unbound

403. Ovulation is caused by a sudden increase in the secretion of which of the following hormones?

a. Estrogen
b. Progesterone
c. LH
d. FSH
e. Prolactin

404. In the following graph of changes in endometrial thickness during a normal 28-day menstrual cycle, the event designated A corresponds most closely to which of the following phases?

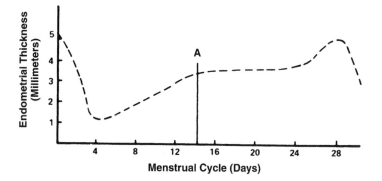

a. The menstrual phase
b. The maturation of the corpus luteum
c. The early proliferative phase
d. The secretory phase
e. Ovulation

405. In a normal pregnancy, human chorionic gonadotropin (hCG) prevents the involution of the corpus luteum that normally occurs at the end of the menstrual cycle. Which of the curves shown below approximates the level of this hormone during pregnancy?

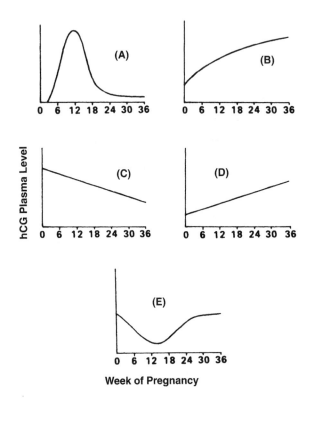

a. A
b. B
c. C
d. D
e. E

406. Activation of hormone-sensitive lipase in adipocytes

a. Causes increased hydrolysis of cholesterol esters
b. Is mediated by a cyclic AMP–dependent protein kinase
c. Is prevented by cortisol
d. Is stimulated by insulin
e. Results in accumulation of monoglycerides and diglycerides in adipocytes

407. Which of the following is a function of Sertoli cells in the seminiferous tubules?

a. Secretion of FSH into the tubular lumen
b. Secretion of testosterone into the tubular lumen
c. Maintenance of the blood-testis barrier
d. Synthesis of estrogen after puberty
e. Expression of surface LH receptors

408. Which of the following is an indication that ovulation has taken place?

a. An increase in serum FSH levels
b. A drop in body temperature
c. An increase in serum LH levels
d. An increase in serum progesterone levels
e. An increase in serum estrogen levels

409. Which of the following hormones is involved in the ejection of milk from a lactating mammary gland?

a. Prolactin
b. FSH
c. LH
d. Growth hormone
e. Oxytocin

410. Plasma levels of calcium can be increased most rapidly by the direct action of PTH on which of the following?

a. Kidney
b. Intestine
c. Thyroid gland
d. Bones
e. Skeletal musculature

411. Which of the following is a correct statement about human growth hormone?

a. It is synthesized in the hypothalamus
b. It stimulates production of somatomedins by the liver
c. Its release is stimulated by somatostatin
d. It causes a decrease in lipolysis
e. It is deficient in acromegaly

412. Which of the following is true about the actions of glucagon?

a. It stimulates glycogenolysis in muscle
b. It inhibits insulin secretion
c. It stimulates gluconeogenesis in the liver
d. It inhibits adenyl cyclase
e. It inhibits phospholipase C

413. The actions of insulin include which of the following?

a. Converting glycogen to glucose
b. Stimulating gluconeogenesis
c. Increasing plasma amino acid concentration
d. Enhancing potassium entry into cells
e. Reducing urine formation

414. The secretion of ACTH is correctly described in which of the following statements?

a. It shows circadian rhythm in humans
b. It is decreased during periods of stress
c. It is inhibited by aldosterone
d. It is stimulated by glucocorticoids
e. It is stimulated by epinephrine

415. Injection of thyroid hormone into a human subject will

a. Decrease the rate of oxygen consumption
b. Increase muscle protein synthesis
c. Decrease the need for vitamins
d. Increase the plasma concentration of cholesterol
e. Decrease the rate of lipolysis

416. Which of the following is an effect of primary hyperaldosteronism (Conn's syndrome)?

a. Hypertension
b. Hyperkalemia
c. Decreased extracellular fluid volume
d. Increased concentrating ability of the kidney
e. Increased hematocrit

417. Hyperparathyroidism decreases the plasma levels of

a. Phosphate
b. Sodium
c. Calcium
d. Potassium
e. Calcitonin

418. Adrenalectomy is associated with which of the following?

a. Hyperglycemia with decreased insulin sensitivity
b. Increased mobilization and utilization of fatty tissues
c. Augmented water excretion by the kidneys and sodium loss in the urine
d. Improved resistance to infection or shock
e. Euphoria

419. Hyperthyroidism is characterized by which of the following?

a. Anorexia
b. Increased basal metabolic rate
c. Bradycardia
d. Increased weight gain
e. Decreased sweating

420. Insulin-independent glucose uptake occurs in which of the following sites?

a. Adipose tissue
b. Cardiac muscle
c. Skeletal muscle
d. The brain
e. The uterus

421. Which one of the following statements is correct?

a. About 100 mg of iron is absorbed per day
b. Iron is absorbed rapidly from the small intestine
c. Iron is transported in the blood bound to transferrin
d. In general, iron must be oxidized from the ferrous to the ferric state for efficient absorption

422. A person with hypothyroidism would exhibit which of the following symptoms?

a. Tachycardia
b. Increased metabolic rate
c. Heat intolerance
d. Sleepiness
e. Decreased body mass index

423. Assuming a regular menstrual cycle of 28 to 30 days, ovulation would be expected to occur between

a. Days 6 and 8
b. Days 10 and 12
c. Days 14 and 16
d. Days 18 and 20
e. Days 22 and 24

424. Secretion of growth hormone is stimulated by which of the following?

a. Increased plasma glucose levels
b. Deep sleep
c. Free fatty acids
d. Somatostatin
e. Hyperglycemia

425. The uptake of triglycerides into adipose tissue from plasma lipoproteins

a. Is regulated by the activity of lipoprotein lipase
b. Is increased by catecholamines
c. Is decreased by glucose
d. Is decreased by insulin
e. Requires receptor-mediated endocytosis

426. Implantation of the zygote in the uterine wall

a. Precedes formation of the zona pellucida
b. Involves infiltration of the endometrium by the syncytiotrophoblast
c. Occurs 3 to 5 days after fertilization
d. Occurs when the embryo consists of approximately 128 cells
e. Is inhibited by secretion of progesterone from the corpus luteum

427. Biological actions of estrogens include which of the following?

a. Inhibition of follicular growth
b. Delayed bone loss at menopause
c. Increased glucose tolerance
d. Decreased serum LDL cholesterol
e. Decreased progesterone receptors

428. Which of the following hormones is primarily responsible for development of ovarian follicles prior to ovulation?

a. Chorionic gonadotropin
b. Estradiol
c. Follicle-stimulating hormone
d. Luteinizing hormone
e. Progesterone

429. Thyroid hormones

a. Are short-acting hormones
b. Have no effect on basal metabolic activity
c. Are stored in extracellular sites
d. Exist in the plasma primarily as free hormones
e. Increase the metabolic activity of the brain

430. Melatonin

a. Is synthesized in the anterior pituitary gland
b. Regulates skin pigmentation in humans
c. Secretion is increased by darkness
d. Secretion is inhibited by norepinephrine from the sympathetic nervous system
e. Is synthesized from the amino acid L-arginine

431. Insulin deficiency leads to which of the following?

a. Increased cellular uptake of glucose
b. Decreased intracellular α-glycerophosphate in liver and fat cells
c. Enhanced glucose uptake and use except by brain tissue
d. Decreased fatty acid release from adipose tissue
e. Indirect depression in use of glucose by excess fatty acids in the blood

432. The islets of Langerhans

a. Are found primarily in the head of the pancreas
b. Constitute approximately 30% of the pancreatic weight
c. Contain six distinct endocrine cell types
d. Have a meager blood supply
e. Secrete insulin and glucagon

433. Which of the following statements about progesterone is true?

a. Progesterone is secreted by the corpus luteum
b. Progesterone secretion by the placenta increases at week 6 of gestation
c. Progesterone plasma levels increase during the menses
d. Progesterone plasma levels remain constant after implantation
e. Progesterone plasma levels decrease subsequent to ovulation

434. The anti-inflammatory effect of cortisol treatment is thought to be due to which of the following?

a. Increased capillary membrane permeability
b. Increased formation of leukotrienes
c. Increased release of pyrogen from granulocytes
d. Activation of phospholipase A_2
e. Stabilization of cellular lysosomal membranes

435. Administration of estrogens in women will

a. Limit the growth of ovarian follicles
b. Produce cyclic changes in the vagina and endometrium
c. Cause cervical mucus to become thicker and more acidic
d. Retard ductal proliferation in the breast

436. Which of the following is the principal androgen responsible for transforming undifferentiated fetal external genitalia into male external genitalia?

a. Müllerian-inhibiting substance
b. Androstenedione
c. Dihydrotestosterone
d. Testosterone
e. Androsterone

437. Which one of the following statements about growth and development is correct?

a. Thyroid hormones are essential for normal growth during puberty
b. Linear growth ceases earlier in boys than in girls
c. Serum IGF-1 levels decrease throughout childhood
d. Growth hormone is essential for prenatal linear growth
e. Prepubertal growth rates are constant throughout the year

438. Which one of the following hormones initiates a biological effect by activation of cell membrane receptors?

a. Progesterone
b. Estrogens
c. Cortisol
d. Epinephrine
e. Thyroxine

439. Which of the following hormones interacts with a cytoplasmic receptor and then localizes in the nucleus and directs protein and nucleotide synthesis?

a. Thyrotropin-releasing hormone
b. Epinephrine
c. Luteinizing hormone
d. Cortisol
e. Insulin

440. Which of the following hormones is responsible for stimulating milk letdown?

a. Oxytocin
b. Progesterone
c. Estradiol
d. Insulin
e. Prolactin

441. A patient with chronic asthma is started on glucocorticoid therapy. The treatment may result in bone loss because glucocorticoids

a. Inhibit bone formation
b. Increase calcium absorption from the GI tract
c. Increase osteoblast growth
d. Inhibit bone resorption
e. Suppress vitamin D activation

442. Hormone replacement therapy is being considered for a 55-year-old woman undergoing menopause. Which of the following is a benefit of the therapy?

a. A return to normal menstrual cycle pattern
b. Hot flashes
c. A reduced risk of stroke
d. Increased risk of osteoporosis

443. Which of the following is the hallmark of pheochromocytoma?

a. Hypertension
b. Hypoglycemia
c. Dry skin
d. Lethargy
e. Bradycardia

444. Plasma catecholamine levels will increase when

a. Blood pressure increases
b. Anxiety increases
c. Blood volume increases
d. Blood glucose increases
e. Moving from a standing to a supine position

445. Cortisol administration to a patient with adrenal insufficiency will

a. Increase insulin sensitivity in muscle
b. Enhance wound healing
c. Increase corticotropin-releasing hormone secretion
d. Increase ACTH secretion
e. Increase gluconeogenesis

446. The signs and symptoms of a patient with primary adrenal insufficiency include which one of the following?

a. Pallor
b. Low ACTH levels
c. High cortisol levels
d. Hyperkalemia
e. Hypertension

447. Which one of the following statements about semen is correct?

a. The bulk of semen volume is contributed by the prostate gland
b. It prevents sperm capacitation
c. It buffers vaginal acidity
d. It activates sperm motility in the male tract
e. Sperm counts have increased over the last 20 years

448. Which of the following statements about atrial natriuretic factor is correct?

a. Secretion increases when central venous pressure increases
b. It constricts afferent renal arterioles
c. It acts only on the distal nephron to increase urine flow
d. It enhances antidiuretic hormone (ADH) secretion
e. Secretion is stimulated by hyponatremia

449. A patient is diagnosed with acromegaly. Patients with this disease typically have which of the following signs?

a. Decreased gluconeogenesis
b. Hypoglycemia
c. Insulin resistance
d. Decreased protein synthesis
e. Decreased lipolysis

450. Prolactin secretion is tonically suppressed in nonpregnant women by which of the following hormones?

a. Estrogen
b. Progesterone
c. Dopamine
d. FSH
e. LH

451. A woman tests positive for pregnancy. In order for the pregnancy to proceed uneventfully, which of the following must occur?

a. The corpus luteum must secrete progesterone to sustain the endometrium
b. The pituitary must secrete hCG to maintain the corpus luteum
c. The pituitary must secrete prolactin to sustain the placenta
d. The placenta must secrete FSH to maintain ovarian function
e. The placenta must secrete LH to maintain ovarian function

452. Symptoms of hypoglycemia develop when the plasma glucose concentration falls to between 45 and 50 mg% and may include which of the following symptoms?

a. Dry skin
b. Bradycardia
c. Insomnia
d. Loss of fine motor skills
e. Satiety

453. Radiation treatment for a pituitary tumor in an 8-year-old boy results in the complete loss of pituitary function. As a result, the child is likely to experience which of the following symptoms?

a. Hypothyroidism and goiter
b. Increased ACTH
c. Absent sexual maturation
d. Accelerated growth spurts
e. Increased TSH levels

454. Which one of the following statements is correct?

a. Thyroid hormones are highly soluble in water
b. Secretion of TSH is regulated primarily by the pituitary level of T_3
c. TSH is secreted from the posterior pituitary
d. TSH initiates thyroid hormone secretion via activation of nuclear receptors in thyroid gland cells
e. T_4 is the physiologically active hormone

455. Maternal physiology changes dramatically throughout pregnancy. Which one of the following changes would be expected?

a. Reduced circulating gonadotrophin levels
b. Increased conversion of glucose to glycogen
c. Hypercapnia
d. Increased hematocrit

456. Which one of the following conditions experienced by pregnant women may be due to the effects of pregnancy?

a. Increased incidence of heartburn
b. Decreased facial acne
c. Increased gastric emptying leading to intestinal cramping and diarrhea
d. Decreased afterload
e. Increased cardiac output

457. Which one of the following is associated with prolonged fasting (3 or more days)?

a. Decreased lipolysis
b. Increased urinary excretion of nitrogen
c. Decreased gluconeogenesis
d. Increased glucose utilization by the brain
e. Increased secretion of insulin

Endocrine Physiology

Answers

387. The answer is a. *(Boron, pp 1010–1013. Guyton, pp 846–849.)* It is thought that the secretion of antidiuretic hormone (ADH)—also called arginine vasopressin (AVP)—and oxytocin by the neurohypophysis is regulated in the hypothalamic supraoptic and paraventricular nuclei, respectively. This hypothalamic control of secretion of pituitary hormone (inhibitory as well as releasing) in the case of the neurohypophysis is by direct neural connection, and, in the case of the adenohypophysis, by humoral factors conveyed by a microcirculation known as the hypothalamic-hypophyseal portal system.

388. The answer is e. *(Boron, pp 1090–1095. Guyton, pp 906–908.)* PTH, secreted by the chief cells of the parathyroid gland, is essential for life. The secretion of PTH is inversely related to the circulating levels of ionized calcium. PTH has a direct effect on bone, involving cAMP changes in osteoblast and osteocyte permeability. It also increases calcium absorption from the gut, although that effect is the result of PTH-mediated increases in renal 1,2,5-dihydroxy-cholecalciferol.

389. The answer is b. *(Boron, pp 1128–1134.)* Sertoli cells are required for germ cell mitotic and meiotic activity. Throughout the reproductive life of the human male, 100 to 200 million sperm are produced daily. Of critical importance to the hormonal regulation of spermatogenesis are the pulsatile release of GRH and the subsequent involvement of FSH and LH at their target cells. FSH acts directly on the Sertoli cells of the seminiferous tubules to initiate mitotic and meiotic activity of germ cells. LH effects are thought to be mediated via stimulation of testosterone secretion by the Leydig cells.

390. The answer is b. *(Boron, pp 1025–1027.)* Numerous factors serve as a stimulus for growth hormone (GH) release, including hypoglycemia (e.g., insulin administration); moderate-to-severe exercise; stress due to emotional disturbances, illness, and fever; and dopamine agonists such as bromocriptine. GH, also known as somatotropin, is among a group of tropic hormones, including prolactin, ACTH, TSH, LH, and FSH, that are synthesized, stored, and secreted by the endocrine cells of the anterior pituitary. Its release is stimulated by growth hormone–releasing hormone (GHRH) and inhibited by somatostatin.

391–392. The answers are 391-b, 392-c. *(Boron, pp 1178–1180. Guyton, pp 946–950.)* During the first two months of pregnancy, estrogen and progesterone production is primarily the responsibility of the corpus luteum. The placenta serves as the source of the hormones during the remainder of pregnancy. Progesterone is essential to maintain placental implantation, inhibit uterine contractions, and suppress the maternal immune system response to fetal antigens. Estrogens serve to increase the size of the uterus, induce progesterone and oxytocin receptors, stimulate maternal hepatic protein secretion, and promote breast development. Estriol is the major estrogen produced during pregnancy. The production of estrogen and progesterone during gestation requires cooperation between the maternal, placental, and fetal compartments—the fetoplacental unit.

393. The answer is b. *(Boron, pp 1010–1013.)* Oxytocin is secreted by the posterior pituitary and is involved in lactation and parturition. The pituitary gland (the hypophysis) is located just beneath the hypothalamus and is connected to the hypothalamus by the infundibulum. It is a compound gland consisting of an anterior lobe (adenohypophysis) and a neural, or posterior, lobe. The anterior pituitary secretes six physiologically important hormones that govern the function of the thyroid (TSH) and adrenal glands (ACTH), the mammary glands (prolactin), and the gonads (FSH, LH) as well as regulate growth (GH).

394. The answer is d. *(Boron, pp 1010–1013.)* Unique among the pituitary hormones, prolactin secretion is tonically inhibited by the hypothalamus. Prolactin is a single-chain protein secreted by the anterior pituitary whose principal physiologic effects involve breast development and milk production. Consistent with its role in lactogenesis, prolactin secretion increases during pregnancy. Dopamine has many characteristics of the hypothalamic inhibitory factor, although it is not found in the hypothalamus.

395. The answer is c. *(Boron, pp 1051–1053. Guyton, pp 869–872.)* Because it lacks 3β-hydroxysteroid dehydrogenase, the enzyme that converts pregnenolone to progesterone (the initial step in both glucocorticoid and mineralocorticoid synthesis), the fetal cortex synthesizes primarily dehydroepiandrosterone. This steroid is released as its sulfate and is metabolized further to estrogen and androgen by the placenta. During fetal life, the adrenal cortex consists of a thin subcapsular rim, which eventually gives rise to the adult cortex, and a thick inner fetal cortex, which constitutes 80% of the gland. This zone undergoes rapid involution after birth.

396. The answer is b. (*Boron, pp 1076–1081. Guyton, pp 886–890.*) Insulin increases glucose uptake by adipocytes. Transport of glucose into cells is by facilitated diffusion. Insulin increases the number of transporters available for glucose uptake in many cells, including adipocytes, skeletal, and cardiac muscle, and some smooth muscle. Insulin does not enhance glucose transport into brain cells, intestinal mucosal cells, or renal tubular epithelial cells.

397. The answer is d. (*Guyton, pp 878–879.*) Cortisol is the only hormone that has a diurnal variation, as shown in the graph accompanying the question. Plasma cortisol levels rise sharply during sleep, peaking soon after awakening, and sinking to a low level approximately 12 h later. This pattern is intimately related to the secretory rhythm of ACTH, which governs—and, in turn, is partly governed by—plasma concentration of cortisol.

398. The answer is c. (*Guyton, pp 929–933.*) Ovulation takes place just after the peak of the luteinizing hormone (LH) and estrogen curves, which occurs on approximately the fourteenth day of the menstrual cycle. Although FSH is primarily responsible for follicular maturation within the ovary, LH is necessary for final follicular maturation; without it, ovulation cannot take place. Both estrogen, following a sharp preovulatory rise in plasma concentration, and progesterone are secreted in abundance by the postovulatory corpus luteum.

399. The answer is b. (*Boron, pp 1037–1038. Guyton, pp 858–864.*) The thyroid gland stores iodide primarily as thyroglobulin. The thyroid gland has a specialized active transport system that very efficiently traps iodide from circulating blood and can accumulate iodide against a large concentration gradient. Within the thyroid, the iodide rapidly undergoes organification by which it is oxidized and covalently linked to tyrosine residues in thyroglobulin. The iodinated tyrosine residues gradually become coupled to form thyroxine, the major secretion product of the thyroid.

400. The answer is d. (*Guyton, pp 929–933.*) There is a marked increase in progesterone secretion following ovulation. Almost all the progesterone secreted in nonpregnant women is secreted by the corpus luteum. Secretion of both progesterone and estrogen is controlled by luteinizing hormone (LH) released by the adenohypophysis, and LH release itself is under the direction of a hypothalamic releasing factor.

401. The answer is b. (*Boron, pp 1146, 1155–1160. Guyton, pp 858–864.*) Thyroxine is the main thyroid hormone entering the circulation and constitutes approximately 95% of active plasma thyroid hormone; the percentage remaining is almost entirely triiodothyronine, which, although more potent than thyroxine, has a more transient presence. Thyroglobulin is the principal storage form of thyroid hormone within the gland, and very little is released into the blood. Thyrotropin (TSH) and long-acting thyroid stimulator (LATS) both stimulate thyroid hormone production and growth of the thyroid gland.

402. The answer is e. (*Guyton, pp 858–860.*) Only the free unbound form of thyroxine is physiologically active. Circulating thyroxine can be bound to albumin, thyroxine-binding prealbumin (TBPA), or thyroxine-binding globulin (TBG). Most thyroxine is bound, and, despite the large available pool of albumin, most of it is bound to TBG. This reflects the relatively greater affinity of TBG for thyroxine.

403. The answer is c. (*Boron, pp 1156–1160.*) Ovulation is caused by a sudden increase in LH secretion. Both LH and FSH blood levels increase during the follicular phase of the menstrual cycle and reach peak blood levels prior to ovulation. Estrogen levels follow a similar pattern during the follicular phase. The physiological signal for ovulation is a surge in LH blood levels. Under the influence of LH, thecal and granulosa cells become the luteal cells of the corpus luteum. Progesterone production by the corpus luteum increases significantly. Estrogen levels also increase, but do not reach the levels achieved during the follicular phase.

404. The answer is e. *(Boron, pp 1156–1162.)* Ovulation occurs at point A on the graph. In response to estrogen secretion by the ovary, the endometrial lining of the uterus undergoes proliferation of both glandular epithelium and supporting stroma during the first 10 to 14 days of the menstrual cycle. Following ovulation, the glands begin to secrete mucus and the stroma undergoes pseudodecidual reaction in preparation for potential pregnancy. When ovulation is not followed by implantation of a fertilized ovum, progesterone secretion declines as the corpus luteum involutes, and the endometrial lining is almost completely shed during menses.

405. The answer is a. *(Boron, pp 1178. Guyton, pp 948–950.)* Human chorionic gonadotropin (hCG) begins to appear in the maternal blood approximately 6 to 8 days following ovulation, upon implantation of the fertilized ovum in the endometrium. The secretion of hCG is essential to prevent involution of the corpus luteum and to stimulate secretion of progesterone and estrogens, which continues until the placenta becomes large enough to secrete sufficient quantities of those hormones. Following a peak at 7 to 9 weeks, hCG secretion gradually declines to a low level by 20 weeks' gestation.

406. The answer is b. *(Guyton, pp 786–787.)* Hormone-sensitive lipase is a cytoplasmic enzyme in adipocytes that catalyzes the complete hydrolysis of triglyceride to fatty acids and glycerol. It is activated by a cyclic AMP–dependent protein kinase that phosphorylates the enzyme, converting it to its active form. Because no accumulation of monoglycerides or diglycerides is detected in adipocytes following the action of hormone-sensitive lipase, it is the initial hydrolysis of triglyceride to fatty acid and diglyceride that is the rate-limiting step. Hormone-sensitive lipase is sensitive to several hormones in vitro, but it appears to be regulated in vivo primarily by epinephrine and glucagon, which activate it by increasing cyclic AMP, and insulin, which inhibits it by preventing cyclic AMP–dependent phosphorylation. Cortisol enhances lipolysis indirectly by promoting increased enzyme synthesis.

407. The answer is c. *(Boron, pp 1127–1133.)* The Sertoli cells rest on a basal lamina and form a layer around the periphery of the seminiferous tubules. They are attached to each other by specialized junctional complexes that limit the movement of fluid and solute molecules from the interstitial space and blood to the tubular lumen, and thus form a blood-testis barrier that provides an immunologically privileged environment for sperm maturation. Sertoli cells are intimately associated with developing spermatozoa and play a major role in germ-cell maturation. They secrete a variety of serum proteins and an androgen-binding protein into the tubular fluid in response to FSH and testosterone stimulation. Testosterone is synthesized and secreted by the interstitial Leydig cells. Estrogen is produced in small amounts by the Sertoli cells before puberty.

408. The answer is d. *(Boron, pp 1156–1162.)* Progesterone production by the corpus luteum increases significantly at the time of ovulation. Both LH and FSH blood levels increase during the follicular phase of the menstrual cycle and reach peak blood levels prior to ovulation. Estrogen levels follow a similar pattern during the follicular phase. The physiologic signal for ovulation is a surge in LH blood levels. Under the influence of LH, thecal and granulosa cells become the luteal cells of the corpus luteum. Estrogen levels also increase, but do not reach the levels achieved during the follicular phase. Progesterone affects the set point for thermoregulation and increases body temperature approximately 0.5°F.

409. The answer is e. *(Guyton, pp 954–956.)* A combined neurogenic and hormonal reflex involving oxytocin, a posterior pituitary hormone, causes the actual ejection ("let-down") of milk from breast tissue. Although estrogen and progesterone are essential for the physical development of breast tissue during pregnancy, both hormones inhibit milk secretion. Milk secretion is regulated by prolactin, a pituitary hormone secreted throughout pregnancy and after parturition. Adequate amounts of growth hormone are required to provide the nutrients that are essential for milk production by breast tissue. Suckling on breast tissue is the stimulus that leads to milk secretion.

410. The answer is d. *(Boron, pp 1090–1095. Guyton, pp 906–909.)* PTH increases plasma calcium levels primarily by mobilizing bone calcium. The main function of the parathyroid gland is to maintain a constant ionized calcium level in the extracellular fluid. To do this, PTH stimulates increased plasma calcium levels, chiefly by mobilizing calcium from bones. Although PTH can also increase renal tubular reabsorption of calcium and intestinal absorption of calcium, these effects depend on adequate dietary ingestion of calcium and thus occur more slowly.

411. The answer is b. (*Boron, pp 1023–1029.*) GH increases the production and release of somatomedins from the liver. These peptides have a multitude of effects on the body and promote growth of organs, bones, and lean body mass. Human growth hormone (GH) is a peptide that is synthesized and released from the anterior pituitary. Its release is stimulated by growth hormone–releasing hormone (GHRH) and inhibited by somatostatin. Both of these peptides are synthesized and released by the hypothalamus and their releases are regulated by multiple feedback loops. GH has the direct effect on adipose tissue of decreasing glucose uptake and increasing lipolysis.

412. The answer is c. (*Boron, pp 1081–1082. Guyton, pp 891–893.*) The primary action of glucagon is to increase blood glucose concentration, which it accomplishes by promoting gluconeogenesis and glycogenolysis in the liver but not in muscle. These effects are mediated by cyclic AMP, which is produced by hepatic adenyl cyclase following interaction of glucagon with its plasma membrane receptor. Interaction of glucagon with different hepatic plasma membrane receptors activates phospholipase C, which results in a rise in concentration of intracellular Ca^{2+}, which further stimulates glycogenolysis. Although glucagon opposes the action of insulin, it does not directly affect insulin secretion.

413. The answer is d. (*Boron, pp 1076–1081. Guyton, pp 884–893.*) One of insulin's major effects is the stimulation of the Na-K pump, which increases potassium entry into cells. Insulin given along with glucose, to prevent hypoglycemia, is often used as a treatment for hyperkalemia. Insulin's major effect on metabolism is the synthesis of proteins and lipids and the storage of glucose as glycogen. Insulin stimulates the uptake of amino acids and glucose by most cells of the body and decreases the rate of gluconeogenesis. Insulin has no effect on urine formation, but in diabetes, when glucose levels increase to a level at which the kidney can no longer reabsorb the filtered glucose, glucose acts as an osmotic diuretic and increases the formation of urine.

414. The answer is a. (*Boron, pp 1056–1057. Guyton, pp 878–880.*) The secretion of ACTH occurs in several irregular bursts during the day; the peak occurs early in the morning prior to awakening and thus is not due to the stress of arising. This circadian rhythm—maximum secretion in early morning, minimum in the evening—is regulated by the hypothalamus through the secretion of corticotropin-releasing hormone (CRH) into the hypothalamic-hypophyseal portal capillary system. In addition to the basal rhythm, physical or mental stress will lead to increased ACTH secretion within minutes. ACTH is also regulated as a result of feedback inhibition by the hormones whose synthesis it stimulates, such as glucocorticoids. Aldosterone is a mineralocorticoid and is not controlled by ACTH. Epinephrine does not appear to have any effect on ACTH secretion.

415. The answer is b. *(Boron, pp 1076–1081.)* Thyroid hormone affects all aspects of metabolism; it increases calorigenesis in every tissue in the body. The hormone stimulates protein synthesis, which may be directly responsible for a portion of its calorigenic effect. Thyroid hormone affects both synthesis and degradation of lipids; the net effect is a decrease in lipid stores. By increasing the mechanisms by which cholesterol is eliminated from the body, thyroid hormone decreases plasma cholesterol levels. Because of its stimulatory effect on metabolic processes, thyroid hormone increases the demand for coenzymes and vitamins.

416. The answer is b. *(Guyton, p 882.)* The symptoms of primary hyperaldosteronism (Conn's syndrome) develop from chronic excess secretion of aldosterone from the zona glomerulosa of the adrenal cortex. Patients are hypertensive and have an expanded blood volume with a decreased hematocrit. They are not markedly hypernatremic because of a renal escape phenomenon. Patients are severely depleted of potassium and, as a consequence, suffer kidney damage, with a resulting loss in concentrating ability.

417. The answer is a. *(Guyton, pp 910–911.)* Hyperparathyroidism decreases plasma phosphate levels. Parathyroid hormone (PTH) is essential for maintaining plasma calcium and phosphate levels. It is released in response to decreased plasma calcium and acts to increase calcium reabsorption and phosphate excretion.

418. The answer is a. *(Guyton, pp 880–882.)* Adrenalectomy leads to diuresis and natriuresis. Removal of the adrenal glands produces the clinical picture known as Addison's disease, a disorder associated with deprivation of adrenocortical hormones. Thus, a lack of glucocorticoids diminishes the body's ability to synthesize glucose by gluconeogenesis. Severe mineralocorticoid deprivation produces grave fluid and electrolyte disturbances as an ultimate consequence of impaired sodium reabsorption, excessive potassium plasma levels, and acidosis.

419. The answer is b. (*Guyton, pp 861–864.*) Hyperthyroidism can increase the basal metabolic rate 60 to 100% above normal. Thyroid hormone causes nuclear transcription of large numbers of genes in virtually all cells of the body. The result is a generalized increase in functional cell activity and metabolism. The increased metabolic activity of patients with hyperthyroidism is accompanied by increased food intake. Nevertheless, their body weight decreases. The generalized increase in cellular activity results in increased sweat production and increased heart rate. The latter sign is often used by physicians to determine whether a patient has increased thyroid hormone production.

420. The answer is d. (*Boron, pp 1076–1081. Guyton, pp 886–891.*) Insulin does not promote glucose uptake by most brain cells. Insulin does increase glucose uptake in skeletal muscle, cardiac muscle, smooth muscle, adipose tissue, leukocytes, and the liver. In most insulin-sensitive tissues, insulin acts to promote glucose transport by enhancing facilitated diffusion of glucose down a concentration gradient. In the liver, where glucose freely permeates the cell membrane, glucose uptake is increased as a result of its phosphorylation by glucokinase. Formation of glucose-6-phosphate reduces the intracellular concentration of free glucose and maintains the concentration gradient favoring movement of glucose into the cell.

421. The answer is c. (*Boron, pp 973–974. Guyton, pp 387–388.*) Iron is transported in the blood bound to the beta globulin, transferrin. Excess iron is stored in all cells, but especially in hepatocytes where it combines with apoferritin. The stored form is called ferritin. The rate of iron absorption is extremely slow, with a maximum of only a few milligrams per day. Iron is absorbed primarily in the ferrous form. Therefore, ferrous iron compounds, rather than ferric compounds, are effective in treating iron deficiency.

422. The answer is d. (*Boron, pp 1090–1095.*) Sleepiness is common in patients with hypothyroidism. Hypothyroidism is a condition usually characterized by low levels of T_3 and T_4, owing to atrophy of the thyroid gland. In very rare cases there is resistance to the effects of thyroid hormones. A deficiency of thyroid hormones or their effects results in bradycardia, which is due to decreased sympathetic activity, and a decreased metabolic rate with its associated sleepiness, weight gain, and cold intolerance. Excess thyroid hormone increases metabolic rate, which increases heat production, stimulates the appetite, and causes weight loss even in the face of increased intake of food. Heat intolerance is characteristic of hyperthyroidism.

423. The answer is c. *(Boron, pp 1145–1146. Guyton, pp 929–933.)* In a woman with a menstrual cycle of 28 to 30 days, ovulation generally occurs between days 14 and 16. The menstrual cycle is divided physiologically into three phases. The follicular phase begins with the onset of menses and lasts 9 to 13 days. The ovulatory phase lasts 1 to 3 days and culminates in ovulation. The luteal phase, the most constant phase of the cycle, lasts about 14 days and ends with the onset of menstrual bleeding.

424. The answer is b. *(Boron, pp 1025–1027.)* Deep sleep induces the greatest daily peak in the secretion of growth hormone. Synthesis and secretion of growth hormone by the anterior pituitary is regulated by a variety of metabolic factors, many of which act to alter the balance between release of growth hormone–releasing hormone (GHRH) and somatostatin (SS) from the hypothalamus. Insulin-induced hypoglycemia is a major stimulus for release of growth hormone. Amino acids are also potent stimuli for release of growth hormone, whereas fatty acids are inhibitory. Thyroxine acts directly on pituitary cells to enhance synthesis of growth hormone and is required for the normal responsiveness of the pituitary and hypothalamus to physiologic stimuli.

425. The answer is a. *(Guyton, pp 886–890.)* Triglyceride uptake into adipocytes is regulated by lipoprotein lipase. The uptake of triglycerides into adipose tissue and other tissues from plasma lipoproteins requires hydrolysis of triglyceride to fatty acids and glycerol by an enzyme bound to the endothelial surface, lipoprotein lipase. The activity of this enzyme varies in reciprocal fashion with that of cytoplasmic hormone-sensitive lipase; that is, its activity is enhanced by insulin and glucose and decreased by catecholamines. Lipoprotein lipase is present in nearly every tissue and acts at the capillary surface as it does in adipose tissue. Receptor-mediated endocytosis is important in the turnover of the protein portion of plasma lipoproteins.

426. The answer is b. *(Boron, pp 1171–1176. Guyton, pp 944–946.)* Implantation of a zygote into the uterine wall involves infiltration of the endometrium by the syncytiotrophoblast. Fertilization and early cleavage of the zygote occur in the fallopian tube in the human female. After approximately 3 days, the zygote enters the uterine cavity, where it undergoes additional divisions over a period of 3 to 4 days to form a morula of approximately 60 cells that is transformed into a blastocyst consisting of the yolk sac and embryo. Enzymatic digestion of the zona pellucida and infiltration of the endometrium by the syncytiotrophoblast, which forms the outer layer of the blastocyst, result in implantation of the blastocyst within the endometrium, where it erodes into maternal vessels. During these early stages of embryogenesis, the endometrium is primed by progesterone secreted by the corpus luteum in the ovary in response to pituitary gonadotropin secretion. After 10 to 15 days, placental gonadotropins maintain the corpus luteum until placental synthesis of progesterone is established at 6 to 8 weeks of gestation.

427. The answer is b. *(Boron, pp 1153–1156. Guyton, pp 912, 933–937.)* Some estrogen receptors are found on osteoblasts and estrogen treatment delays age-related bone loss at menopause. At puberty, estrogens stimulate the growth and development of the female reproductive tract and increase the number of progesterone receptors. The metabolic effects of estrogens include antagonizing the actions of insulin on peripheral tissues and decreasing glucose tolerance. Estrogens also decrease serum cholesterol levels.

428. The answer is c. *(Guyton, pp 937–939.)* Preparation of primordial ovarian follicles for ovulation is the primary function of FSH. FSH stimulates development of the theca and granulose cells of the follicles and promotes the synthesis of estrogens, including estradiol. LH promotes luteinization of the postovulatory follicle and stimulates progesterone secretion by the corpus luteum. During pregnancy, hCG is secreted by the placenta and continues progesterone production.

429. The answer is c. *(Guyton, pp 858–864.)* Thyroglobulin, the storage form of thyroid hormones, is stored extracellularly in follicles lined by thyroid epithelium. Only about 0.02% of the thyroxine and about 0.2% of the triiodothyronine are normally present in plasma in the free form; the rest is bound to thyroxine-binding globulin, thyroxine-binding prealbumin, and albumin. Following injection of thyroxine into a human, the effect on the metabolic rate is not noticeable for 2 to 3 days; then the rate begins to increase progressively and reaches a maximum in 10 to 12 days. Some of the activity persists for up to 2 months. The principal effect of the thyroid hormones is an increase in the metabolic rate of most tissues in the body, with a few exceptions such as brain, retina, testes, spleen, and lungs.

430. The answer is c. *(Guyton, pp 926–928.)* Synthesis and secretion of melatonin are increased in the dark via input from norepinephrine secreted by postganglionic sympathetic neurons. Melatonin is synthesized in the pineal gland from the amino acid tryptophan. Pinealomas (tumors of the pineal gland) that destroy the pineal gland and reduce secretion of melatonin and cause hypothalamic damage may cause precocious puberty by removing the inhibitory effect of melatonin on the pituitary response to gonadotropin-releasing hormone. Melatonin causes amphibian skin to become lighter in color but has no role in the regulation of skin color in humans.

431. The answer is b. *(Boron, pp 1076–1081. Guyton, pp 884–891.)* α-Glycerophosphate is produced in the course of normal use of glucose. In the absence of adequate quantities of α-glycerophosphate—a normal acceptor of free fatty acids in triglyceride synthesis—lipolysis will be the predominant process in adipose tissue. As a result, fatty acids will be released into the blood. The prevailing insulin level is decisive in the selection of substrate by a tissue for the production of energy. Insulin promotes use of carbohydrate, and a lack of the hormone causes use of fat mainly to the exclusion of uptake and use of glucose, except by brain tissue. Indirect depression of use of glucose by excess fatty acids is a result, and not a contributing cause, of increased use of fat.

432. The answer is e. *(Guyton, p 884.)* The islets of Langerhans, which constitute 1 to 2% of the pancreatic weight, secrete insulin, glucagon, somatostatin, and pancreatic polypeptide. Each is secreted from a distinct cell type, A, B, D, and F, respectively. Most islet cells are located in the head or body of the pancreas, and each is well vascularized.

433. The answer is a. *(Boron, pp 1156–1181.)* Progesterone is secreted by the corpus luteum. The plasma level of progesterone is low during the menses and remains low until just prior to ovulation. It rises substantially after ovulation, owing to secretion by the corpus luteum. If fertilization occurs, the corpus luteum continues to secrete progesterone until the placenta develops and begins to produce large amounts of the hormone. The plasma level of progesterone rises steadily throughout pregnancy after the placenta takes over production at about 12 weeks of gestation.

434. The answer is e. *(Boron, pp 1053–1057.)* The anti-inflammatory effects of exogenous cortisol are due to its ability to decrease capillary membrane permeability and probably also to its ability to stabilize lysosomal membranes and decrease the formation of bradykinin. Glucocorticoids inhibit the enzyme phospholipase A_2. This decreases the release of arachidonic acid and the variety of substances produced from it, such as leukotrienes, prostaglandins, thromboxanes, and prostacyclin. Cortisol owes its fever-reducing action to the hormone's ability to decrease the release of pyrogen (interleukin 1) from granulocytes. However, only in massive doses will the hormone achieve the effects described. Endogenous cortisol does not exert significant anti-inflammatory action.

435. The answer is b. *(Boron, pp 1153–1156. Guyton, pp 934–936.)* Estrogens cause the mucus secreted by the cervix to become thinner and more alkaline and to exhibit a fernlike pattern upon drying. The epithelium of the vagina is so sensitive to estrogen action that vaginal smear examination is used for a bioassay of the hormone. Estrogens can stimulate growth of ovarian follicles even in hypophysectomized women and also stimulate growth of the glandular epithelium of the endometrium, the smooth muscle of the uterus, and the uterine vascular system. Growth of the glandular elements of the breast is stimulated by progesterone; growth of the ductal elements is stimulated by estrogen.

436. The answer is c. *(Guyton, pp 922–926.)* Androgens, particularly dihydrotestosterone, are essential for regulation of the external genitalia in males. The fetus develops with multipotential internal and external genitalia. The development of male internal genitalia depends upon the presence of two hormones produced by the fetal testis—progesterone and Müllerian-inhibiting substance. The former stimulates growth and development of Wolffian ducts; the latter stimulates Müllerian duct regression.

DHT-regulated development of external sex characteristics occurs between 9 and 12 weeks of gestation.

437. The answer is a. *(Guyton, pp 850–851.)* Thyroid hormones are essential for normal linear growth and skeletal development. The growth-promoting effects of thyroid hormones occur via a synergistic effect with growth hormone. IGF-1 secretions increase throughout childhood and stimulate cell proliferation and growth in many different cell types, including chondrocytes within growth plates. Linear growth ends earlier in girls than in boys. Growth hormone does not play a significant role in prenatal linear growth. Prepubertal growth evidences seasonal variations, with most growth occurring in the spring and summer.

438. The answer is d. *(Boron, pp 1013–1020. Guyton, pp 840–843.)* Due to their relatively low solubility within the lipid portions of the cell membrane, peptide hormones and catecholamines (epinephrine) must interact with receptors located on the cell membrane. Activation of the receptor is followed by the generation of intracellular second messengers that ultimately mediate the biological response to the hormone. Steroid hormones and thyroid hormones readily pass through the cell surface membrane and interact with intracellular receptors to produce their effects by regulating gene expression within the nucleus.

439. The answer is d. *(Boron, pp 1013–1020.)* Cortisol, like other steroid hormones, diffuses into target cells and interacts with intracellular receptors. The steroid-receptor complex has a high affinity for the steroid-responsive element of DNA. Once bound to DNA, the hormone-receptor complex acts as a transcription factor to regulate gene expression and formation of specific messenger RNAs.

440. The answer is a. *(Boron, pp 1185–1187. Guyton, pp 855–856, 956.)* Oxytocin is a posterior pituitary peptide that promotes contraction of the myoepithelial cells surrounding breast ducts and causes expulsion of milk from lobular alveoli. Secretion of oxytocin is promoted by tactile stimulation of the breast by the nursing infant. It can also be elicited by psychic factors alone, such as the anticipation of nursing brought on by hearing the cry of the hungry infant. This anticipatory secretion of oxytocin may be experienced by the mother as a sensation of milk letdown in which milk appears at the nipple and may be forcibly ejected.

441. The answer is a. *(Boron, pp 1052–1054.)* Glucocorticoid therapy enhances bone loss by inhibiting bone formation. It also increases bone resorption. Glucocorticoids are produced by the adrenal glands and have a broad spectrum of action, particularly as it relates to fuel metabolism, response to injury, and general cell function.

442. The answer is c. *(Boron, pp 1153–1156.)* Estrogen replacement therapy decreases a patient's risk of stroke. Hot flashes, osteoporosis, and increased LDL cholesterol are consequences of estrogen deficiency. Estrogen therapy does not restore a woman's ability to have children.

443. The answer is a. *(Boron, pp 1065. Guyton, pp 872–873.)* The hallmark of pheochromocytoma is either sustained or paroxysmal hypertension. Pheochromocytoma is a rare catecholamine-secreting tumor of the adrenal chromaffin cells. Patients with the disease often have associated episodes of sweating, anxiety or nervousness, palpitations, headache, diaphoresis, and hyperglycemia.

444. The answer is b. *(Guyton, pp 703–705.)* Emotional stress increases circulating catecholamine levels. Circumstances that increase sympathetic nerve input to the adrenal medulla increase catecholamine secretion. Major stressors include decreased intravascular volume or pressure, fear or rage, a change in posture from supine to standing, and hypoglycemia.

445. The answer is e. *(Boron, pp 1049–1057.)* Cortisol is defined as a glucocorticoid because it promotes the conversion of amino acids to glucose (gluconeogenesis). It also decreases glucose uptake by muscle and adipocytes by decreasing the sensitivity of the cells to insulin. The net result is to provide more glucose to non-insulin-requiring cells. Cortisol retards wound healing. It also decreases CRH and ACTH secretion by feedback inhibition.

446. The answer is d. *(Boron, pp 786, 824.)* Patients with primary adrenal insufficiency (Addison's disease) are hyperkalemic due to a deficiency of aldosterone. This is accompanied by hyponatremia and hypotension. Hyperpigmentation occurs due to an increased production of melanin. Lack of cortisol leads to high levels of ACTH.

447. The answer is b. *(Boron, pp 1128–1133.)* Sperm contains chemicals that prevent sperm capacitation, thereby prolonging the viability of the sperm. In addition, the high potassium content of the secretion inhibits sperm motility, further adding to the viability. Sperm is secreted primarily by the seminiferous tubules and the alkaline nature of the secretion buffers the acidity of the vagina. In recent years, the average sperm count has decreased from approximately 100 million/mL of semen to 60 to 70 million/mL of semen.

448. The answer is a. *(Boron, pp 555, 772, 788.)* Atrial natriuretic peptide (ANP) is synthesized, stored, and secreted by cardiac atrial muscle, the latter in response to increased central venous pressure or increased plasma sodium concentrations. ANP increases glomerular filtration by simultaneous dilation of afferent and constriction of efferent renal arterioles. It decreases salt and water reabsorption along the entire length of the kidney. The excretion of water is enhanced by inhibition of ADH.

449. The answer is c. *(Boron, p 1024.)* Patients with acromegaly have insulin resistance. In addition, they evidence increased lipolysis and increased gluconeogenesis due to their high growth hormone levels. The combination of enhanced glucose production and insulin resistance can produce hyperglycemia and diabetes mellitus. Protein synthesis increases to support tissue growth and proliferation.

450. The answer is c. *(Guyton, pp 848–849, 954–956.)* In nonpregnant women, the secretion of prolactin is kept tonically suppressed by secretion of dopamine from the hypothalamus. Prolactin is the main hormone of lactation. Hormone levels increase early in pregnancy due to the influence of estrogens. However, lactation does not occur early in pregnancy because estrogens and progesterone inhibit the interaction of prolactin with receptors located on the alveolar cell membranes. At term, estrogen and progesterone levels decrease and milk production begins usually within three days of delivery.

451. The answer is a. (*Guyton, pp 948–949.*) Continuous secretion of progesterone by the corpus luteum is essential for development of the fetus. During the first trimester, placental production of hCG sustains the corpus luteum and ensures continued progesterone secretion. By the second trimester, progesterone production by the placenta increases to levels sufficient to sustain fetal growth and development.

452. The answer is d. (*Guyton, p 897.*) Hypoglycemia can lead to loss of fine motor skills. Hypoglycemia refers to abnormally low blood glucose levels and is dangerous because glucose is the primary energy source for brain cells. Dysfunction of the nervous system can lead to dizziness, headache, mental confusion, convulsion, and loss of consciousness. Increased sympathetic activity can produce sweating, tachycardia, hunger, and anxiety.

453. The answer is c. (*Guyton, pp 846–853.*) Radiation treatment likely produced panhypopituitarism in the young child. Sexual maturation and growth during development will not occur because of low levels of GH, FSH, LF, ILGF1, TSH and thyroid hormones, and gonadal hormones. The cortisol response to stress is decreased due to low ACTH levels. A goiter cannot develop in the absence of TH.

454. The answer is b. (*Boron, pp 1044–1048.*) Secretion of TSH is regulated primarily by the pituitary levels of T_3. As plasma thyroid hormone levels increase, pituitary T_3 levels rise and lead to inhibition of TSH synthesis and secretion. TSH stimulates thyroid gland function by binding to specific cell membrane receptors and increasing the intracellular levels of cAMP. The thyroid gland secretes thyroxine (T_4) and triiodothyronine (T_3); the latter is the physiologically active hormone. The majority of T_3 is formed in the peripheral tissues by deiodination of T_4.

455. The answer is a. (*Guyton, pp 950–952.*) During pregnancy, the maternal hypothalamic-pituitary axis is suppressed due to high circulating levels of sex hormones. This leads to reduced gonadotrophin levels, and, thus, ovulation does not occur. Additionally, hyperventilation leads to decreased arterial carbon dioxide levels. Increased water retention leads to decreased hematocrit. Maternal use of glucose declines and, as a result, gluconeogenesis increases. Plasma cortisol levels increase as the result of progesterone-mediated displacement from transcortin and its subsequent binding to globulin.

456. The answer is a. (*Guyton, pp 950–951.*) Progesterone-mediated relaxation of lower esophageal sphincter smooth muscle is believed to increase the frequency of esophageal reflux and, thus, the sensation of heartburn. Progesterone may also relax gastric and colonic smooth muscle, resulting in gastroparesis and constipation, respectively. Estrogens cause marked peripheral vasodilation. The resultant decrease in afterload leads to a compensatory increase in cardiac output.

457. The answer is c. (*Berne, pp 807, 814–815, 942.*) With prolonged fasting of 3 days or more, gluconeogenesis is decreased partly due to increased ketogenesis and lipolysis. The increased availability of ketones and fatty acids as a source of fuel for brain cells decreases the demand by the brain for glucose. The decreased gluconeogenesis is reflected in a nitrogen excretion level at or below normal values. Insulin levels decrease beginning as early as 24 h after a meal.

Neurophysiology

Questions

DIRECTIONS: Each question below contains several suggested responses. Select the **one best** response to each question.

458. A 22-year-old man sees his ophthalmologist because it is becoming increasing difficult for him to read the newspaper. His vision problem most likely results from an inability to contract which of the following?

a. The iris
b. The ciliary body
c. The suspensory ligaments
d. The extraocular muscles
e. The pupil

459. A 7-year-old boy is evaluated for stapedectomy because of significant hearing problems. The operation restores the function of the middle ear bones. Which of the following is the primary function of the middle ear bones?

a. To amplify sounds
b. To filter high-frequency sounds
c. To localize a sound
d. To enhance frequency discrimination
e. To protect the ear from load sounds

460. During a voluntary movement, the Golgi tendon organ provides the central nervous system with information about which of the following?

a. The length of the muscle being moved
b. The velocity of the movement
c. The blood flow to the muscle being moved
d. The tension developed by the muscle being moved
e. The change in joint angle produced by the movement

461. Repetitive stimulation of a skeletal muscle fiber will cause an increase in contractile strength because repetitive stimulation causes an increase in which of the following?

a. The duration of cross-bridge cycling
b. The concentration of calcium in the myoplasm
c. The magnitude of the end-plate potential
d. The number of muscle myofibrils generating tension
e. The velocity of muscle contraction

462. A 10-year-old girl with type I diabetes develops a neuropathy limited to sensory neurons with free nerve endings. Quantitative sensory testing will reveal higher-than-normal thresholds for the detection of which of the following?

a. Fine touch
b. Vibration
c. Pressure
d. Temperature
e. Muscle length

463. A 16-year-old boy is brought to the emergency room by ambulance after suffering a concussion during a football game. When he awoke he had difficulty expressing himself verbally but was able to understand and follow commands. His condition is most likely caused by damage to which of the following?

a. The hippocampus
b. The temporal lobe
c. The parietal lobe
d. The limbic system
e. The reticular activating system

464. Depolarization of the hair cells in the cochlea is caused primarily by the flow of which of the following?

a. K^+ into the hair cell
b. Na^+ into the hair cell
c. Cl^- out of the hair cell
d. Ca^{2+} into the hair cell
e. Mg^{2+} into the hair cell

465. Which of the following is the most important role of the gamma motoneurons?

a. Stimulate skeletal muscle fibers to contract
b. Maintain Ia afferent activity during contraction of muscle
c. Generate activity in Ib afferent fibers
d. Detect the length of resting skeletal muscle
e. Prevent muscles from producing too much force

466. Each of the figures in the diagram below illustrates a train of action potentials in response to a sudden limb movement. The sensory neuron encoding the velocity of the limb movement is illustrated by which of the following figures?

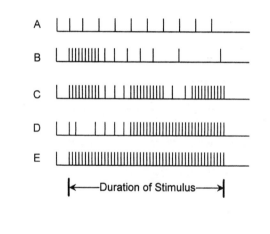

a. A
b. B
c. C
d. D
e. E

467. Which of the following receptors is responsible for measuring the intensity of a steady pressure on the skin surface?

a. Pacinian corpuscle
b. Ruffini ending
c. Merkel's disk
d. Meissner's corpuscle
e. Krause ending

468. A 72-year-old man visits his physician because he finds it difficult to hold his hand steady when painting. Examination reveals a resting tremor and rigidity. The symptoms are relieved by single dose of levodopa. This patient's neurological signs are most likely related to a lesion within which of the following?

a. The vestibular nucleus
b. The substantia nigra
c. The premotor area
d. The caudate nucleus
e. The hippocampus

469. The precentral gyrus and corticospinal tract are essential for which of the following?

a. Vision
b. Olfaction
c. Auditory identification
d. Kinesthesia
e. Voluntary movement

470. A 72-year-old male is evaluated by a physiatrist after a stroke. The patient is observed to suffer from dysmetria and ataxia. These neurological signs are most likely related to a lesion within which of the following regions of the brain?

a. Cerebellum
b. Medulla
c. Cortical motor strip
d. Basal ganglia
e. Eighth cranial nerve

471. A 62-year-old man with a history of hypertension and hyperlipidemia is admitted to the hospital for evaluation after demonstrating signs and symptoms of a stroke. Subsequent CT scans, perceptual tests, and a neurological examination provide evidence for impairment of the otolith pathways. The otolith organs (utricle and saccule) are responsible for which of the following?

a. Producing the vestibular-ocular reflex
b. Detecting the position of the head in space
c. Producing rotary nystagmus
d. Detecting angular acceleration
e. Producing the stretch reflex

472. Which of the reactions in the retinal rods is caused directly by the absorption of light energy?

a. Dissociation of scotopsin and metarhodopsin
b. Decomposition of scotopsin
c. Transformation of 11-cis retinal to all-trans retinal
d. Transformation of metarhodopsin to lumirhodopsin
e. Transformation of vitamin A to retinene

473. Which of the following statements about the cerebrospinal fluid (CSF) is true?

a. It is absorbed by the choroid plexus
b. Its absorption is independent of CSF pressure
c. It circulates in the epidural space
d. It has a lower glucose concentration than plasma
e. It has a higher protein concentration than plasma

474. When a person slowly rotates toward the right,

a. The stereocilia on the hair cells in the right horizontal semicircular canal bend away from the kinocilium
b. Both the left and right eyes deviate toward the left
c. The hair cells in the left horizontal semicircular canal become depolarized
d. The visual image on the retina becomes unfocused
e. The endolymph in the left and right horizontal semicircular canals moves in opposite directions

475. During a normal voluntary movement

a. Large muscle fibers are recruited before small muscle fibers
b. Fast muscle fibers are recruited before slow muscle fibers
c. Weak muscle fibers are recruited before strong muscle fibers
d. Poorly perfused muscle fibers are recruited before richly perfused muscle fibers
e. Anaerobic fibers are recruited before aerobic fibers

476. A 41-year-old man is seen by his physician complaining of "always feeling tired" and having "vivid dreams when he is sleeping." He is referred to the hospital's sleep center for evaluation. He is diagnosed with narcolepsy based on his clinical history and the presence of rapid eye movements (REM) as soon as he falls asleep. Which one of the following signs will be observed when the patient is exhibiting REM sleep?

a. Hyperventilation
b. Loss of skeletal muscle tone
c. Slow but steady heart rate
d. High amplitude EEG wave
e. Decreased brain metabolism

477. A 58-year-old woman goes to her physician because she is having difficulty threading needles. After a thorough physical examination she is diagnosed with presbyopia (old eyes). Her condition is caused by which of the following?

a. Clouding of the vitreous
b. Retinal detachment
c. Ciliary muscle paralysis
d. Stiffening of the lens
e. Degeneration of the macula

478. When light strikes the eye there is an increase in which of the following?

a. The activity of the transducin
b. The amount of transmitter released from the photoreceptors
c. The concentration of all-trans retinal within the photoreceptors
d. The concentration of calcium within the photoreceptors
e. The activity of guanylyl cyclase

479. A 64-year-old female patient is referred to a neurologist because her sister and brother both suffered recent strokes. She is diagnosed with an antiphospholipid antibody syndrome, a condition that causes hypercoagulation, and placed on warfarin. Despite the anticoagulation therapy she develops a thrombotic cerebral infarct, which leads to spasticity of her left wrist, elbow, and knee. The lesion most likely affected which of the following?

a. The corticospinal fibers
b. The vestibulospinal fibers
c. The Ia afferent fibers
d. The corticoreticular fibers
e. The reticulospinal fibers

480. Activation of transducin by light activates an enzyme that

a. Hydrolyzes cGMP
b. Increases the dark current
c. Activates adenylyl cyclase
d. Releases calcium from intracellular stores
e. Depolarizes the membrane

481. A 27-year-old patient with severe vertigo is seen by a neurologist. Examination reveals a positional nystagmus. The lesion producing the nystagmus is most likely within which of the following regions of the brain?

a. The reticular formation
b. The flocculonodular lobe
c. The lateral cerebellum
d. The anterior hypothalamus
e. The cingulate gyrus

482. The alpha rhythm appearing on an electroencephalogram has which of the following characteristics?

a. It produces 20 to 30 waves per second
b. It disappears when a patient's eyes open
c. It is replaced by slower, larger waves during REM sleep
d. It represents activity that is most pronounced in the frontal region of the brain
e. It is associated with deep sleep

Questions 483–484

The image distance of a normal relaxed eye is indicated in the diagram below.

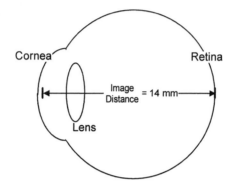

483. The focal length of the eye is

a. 14 mm
b. 15 mm
c. 17 mm
d. 19 mm
e. 21 mm

484. If an object is placed 25 cm away from the eye, the image will be focused on the retina if the refractive power of the eye is increased to which of the following?

a. 64 diopters
b. 68 diopters
c. 70 diopters
d. 72 diopters
e. 75 diopters

485. Tapping the patella tendon elicits a reflex contraction of the quadriceps muscle. During the contraction of the quadriceps muscle,

a. The Ib afferents from the Golgi tendon organ increase their rate of firing
b. The Ia afferents from the muscle spindle increase their rate of firing
c. The alpha motoneurons innervating the extrafusal muscle fibers decrease their rate of firing
d. The gamma motoneurons innervating the intrafusal muscle fibers increase their rate of firing
e. The alpha motoneurons to the antagonistic muscles increase their rate of firing

486. A 59-year-old woman is admitted to the hospital because of agitation and aggression. Three years prior to admission her irregular, flinging movements had become so severe that she could not walk or assist in her own care. She is diagnosed with Huntington's chorea, which is a hereditary disease affecting neurons within which of the following?

a. Anterior cerebellum
b. Subthalamus
c. Substantial nigra
d. Striatum
e. Limbic system

487. Norepinephrine causes contraction of the smooth muscle in which of the following?

a. Bronchioles
b. Pupils
c. Intestine
d. Arterioles
e. Ciliary body

488. A 22-year-old musician visits an otolaryngologist complaining of a ringing in his ear. An audiometry test reveals a high-frequency hearing loss in which the threshold for hearing high-frequency sounds is raised by 1000 times. The patient's hearing loss is

a. 20 decibels
b. 30 decibels
c. 40 decibels
d. 50 decibels
e. 60 decibels

489. If a patient is unable to hear high-frequency sounds, the damage to the basilar membrane is closest to which of the following?

a. Oval window
b. Helicotrema
c. Stria vascularis
d. Modiolus
e. Spiral ganglion

490. A 3-month-old baby is brought to her pediatrician for a check up. Stroking the plantar surface of the foot produces a reflex extension of the large toe rather than the expected flexion. The Babinski sign elicited by the physician indicates damage to which of the following?

a. Spinal cord
b. Brainstem
c. Cerebellum
d. Basal ganglia
e. Pyramids

491. A 41-year-old man complains to his physician about jet lag whenever he flies long distances to meetings. Melatonin is prescribed as a way to reset his circadian rhythm. The circadian rhythm is controlled by which of the following?

a. Paraventricular nucleus
b. Ventromedial nucleus
c. Arcuate nucleus
d. Lateral nucleus
e. Suprachiasmatic nucleus

492. Presynaptic inhibition in the central nervous system affects the firing rate of alpha motoneurons by

a. Increasing the chloride permeability of the presynaptic nerve ending
b. Decreasing the potassium permeability of the alpha motoneuron
c. Decreasing the frequency of action potentials by the presynaptic nerve ending
d. Increasing (hyperpolarizing) the membrane potential of the alpha motoneuron
e. Increasing the amount of the neurotransmitter released by the presynaptic nerve ending

493. Which of the following events accompanies the rapid voluntary flexion of the arm?

a. An increase in the activity of the Ia afferent fibers from the biceps (the agonist)
b. A decrease in the activity of the Ib afferent fibers from the biceps (the agonist)
c. An increase in the activity of the Ia afferent fibers from the triceps (the antagonist)
d. A decrease in the activity of the Ib afferent fibers from the triceps (the antagonist)
e. An increase in the activity of the alpha motoneurons to the triceps (the antagonist)

494. The sympathetic response in a "fight or flight" reaction causes a decrease in which of the following?

a. The arterial blood pressure
b. The diameter of the pupil
c. The resistance of the airways
d. The blood glucose concentration
e. The heart rate

495. A 62-year-old woman is referred to a neurologist by her family physician because of a recent loss of initiative, lethargy, memory problems, and a loss of vision. She is diagnosed with primary hypothyroidism and referred to an endocrinologist for treatment of her thyroid problem and to a neurophthalmologist for visual field evaluation. Which one of the following visual field defects is most likely to be found?

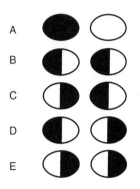

a. A
b. B
c. C
d. D
e. E

496. A 29-year-old woman who complains of slowly progressive loss of vision on her right side affecting both eyes is seen by her neurologist. A CT scan demonstrates a high-density space-occupying lesion. The lesion produces the visual field defect by compressing which of the following?

a. The right lateral geniculate
b. The left optic nerve
c. The right visual cortex
d. The optic chiasm
e. The left optic tract

497. The pain produced by ischemia is poorly localized and throbbing, whereas pain from a needle stick is well localized and sharp. Which of the following comparisons of ischemic and needle stick pain is correct?

a. Ischemic pain sensory fibers are classified as A delta (AD) sensory fibers
b. Ischemic pain is produced by overstimulating somatic touch receptors
c. Ischemic pain is transmitted to the brain through the neospinothalamic tract
d. Ischemic pain receptors quickly adapt to a painful stimulus
e. Ischemic pain sensory fibers terminate within the substantia gelatinosa of the spinal cord

498. A 17-year-old boy is admitted to the hospital with a traumatic brain injury, sustained when he fell off his motorcycle. He develops a fever of 39°C, which is unrelated to an infection or inflammation. The fever is most likely due to a lesion of which of the following?

a. The lateral hypothalamus
b. The arcuate nucleus
c. The posterior nucleus
d. The paraventricular nucleus
e. The anterior hypothalamus

499. In which one of the following sensory systems does stimulation cause the receptor cell to hyperpolarize?

a. Vision
b. Hearing
c. Taste
d. Touch
e. Smell

500. A 29-year-old man is brought to the emergency room after a traffic accident causing a traumatic brain injury. Within several hours he begins eating objects such as paper, is unable to maintain attention, and displays increased sexual activity. He is diagnosed with Klüver-Bucy syndrome, which is produced by bilateral lesions of which of the following regions of the brain?

a. Temporal lobe
b. Hypothalamus
c. Olfactory lobe
d. Hippocampus
e. Cingulate gyrus

Neurophysiology

Answers

458. The answer is b. *(Baron, pp 332–334. Guyton, p 570.)* Contracting the ciliary body increases the refractive power of the eye for near vision. When the ciliary muscle contracts, it pulls the suspensory ligaments toward the cornea, which permits the lens causes the lens surface to bulge, increasing its refractive power. The muscles of the iris control the size of the pupils, and the extraocular muscles control the position of the eye in the socket.

459. The answer is a. *(Baron, pp 347–348. Guyton 602–603, 612.)* When sound waves pass from air to water, most of the energy contained in the sound stimulus is lost. Because the auditory receptors within the inner ear are bathed in liquid, most of the energy in the sound stimulus could be lost as the sound travels from air to water. The bones of the middle ear significantly reduce the amount of loss by amplifying the sound stimulus. Audiologists refer to this amplification phenomenon as impedance matching. Sound localization is carried out by the central nervous system (CNS), which integrates information from both ears. Frequency discrimination is a function of the basilar membrane. The stapedius and tensor tympani muscles protect the ear from loud sounds.

460. The answer is d. *(Baron, 357–358. Guyton, pp 628–629.)* The Golgi tendon organ (GTO) is located in the tendon of skeletal muscles and therefore is in series with the muscle. Each time the muscle contracts, the GTO organ is stretched in proportion to the tension developed by the muscle. The Ib afferent fibers (which innervate the GTO) produce a train of action potentials with a frequency that is in proportion to the deformation of the GTO. The muscle length and speed of shortening are sent to the CNS by Ia afferents that innervate the intrafusal fibers within muscle spindles.

461. The answer is a. *(Baron, pp 249–250. Guyton, p 76.)* Each time a skeletal muscle fiber is stimulated by an alpha motoneuron, enough Ca^{2+} is released from its sarcoplasmic reticulum (SR) to fully activate all the troponin within the muscle. Therefore, every cross bridge can contribute to the generation of tension. However, the transmission of force from the cross bridges to the tendon (or bone or measuring device) does not occur until the series elastic component (SEC) of the muscle is stretched. Repetitive firing increases the amount of SEC stretch by maintaining cross-bridge cycling for a longer period of time. Repetitive firing increases neither the concentration of Ca^{2+} within the myoplasm, the number of myofibrils that are activated, nor the magnitude of the end-plate potential. Because all of the cross bridges are activated each time a skeletal muscle fiber is activated, an increase in Ca^{2+} concentration would have no effect on muscle strength.

462. The answer is d. *(Baron, pp 352–357. Guyton, pp 561–563.)* Free nerve endings contain receptors for temperature, pain, and crude touch. However, fine touch, pressure, and vibration are detected by nerve endings contained within specialized capsules that transmit the stimulus to the sensory receptors. Muscle length is encoded by the primary nerve endings of Ia fibers, which are located on intrafusal fibers within the muscle spindle.

463. The answer is b. *(Guyton, pp 669–671.)* Aphasia is a language disorder in which a person is unable to properly express or understand certain aspects of written or spoken language. It is caused by lesions to the language centers of the brain, which, for the majority of persons, are located within the left hemisphere in the portions of the temporal and frontal lobes known as Wernicke's and Broca's areas, respectively. Language disorders caused by memory loss, which could be the result of a hippocampal lesion, are not classified as aphasias.

464. The answer is a. *(Boron, pp 343–345. Guyton, pp 606–607.)* When the hair cells are bent, K^+ selective channels open, K^+ flows into the cell, and the cell depolarizes. This unusual situation occurs because the apical surface of the hair cells, on which the stereocilia are located, is bathed in endolymph, which contains a high concentration of K^+. Moreover, the endolymph is positively charged with respect to the perilymph, which surrounds the basal lateral portion of the hair cell. Because the intracellular concentration of K^+ is similar to the extracellular concentration of K^+, the electrical gradient determines the direction of K^+ flow. Because the endolymph is positively charged and the intracellular fluid is negatively charged, K^+ flows into the cell.

465. The answer is b. *(Boron, pp 357–358, 362–363. Guyton, pp 624–627.)* The gamma motoneurons innervate the intrafusal fibers of the muscle spindles. When a skeletal muscle contracts, the intrafusal muscle fiber becomes slack and the Ia afferents stop firing. By stimulating the intrafusal muscle fibers during a contraction, the gamma motoneurons prevent the intrafusal muscle fibers from becoming slack and thus maintain Ia firing during the contraction.

466. The answer is b. (*Rhoades, pp 352–354. Guyton, pp 531–533.*) The Ia afferents, which innervate the muscle spindles, have a phasic and tonic component. Part **B** illustrates their response to a sudden movement of a limb. The high-frequency burst of action potentials encodes the velocity of the initial movement, whereas the steady firing encodes the position of the limb when the movement is completed. Parts **A** and **C** illustrate the behavior of a tonic receptor, which discharges at the same rate for as long as the stimulus is present.

467. The answer is b. (*Boron, pp 352–355. Guyton pp 528–529, 541.*) The Ruffini ending is a tonic receptor that produces a train of action potentials proportional to the intensity of pressure applied to the skin. The Pacinian corpuscle is a very rapidly adapting receptor that fires once or twice in response to skin deformation. It can produce a continuous train of action potentials if the stimulus is repetitively applied and withdrawn. Therefore, the Pacinian corpuscle is used to encode vibration.

468. The answer is b. (*Boron, 273–274, 301–302. Guyton, pp 657–660.*) Parkinson's disease is characterized by resting tremor rigidity and akinesia. It is caused by destruction of the dopamine secreting neurons within the substantia nigra. Levo (L)-dopa is a precursor for dopamine. L-dopa, rather than dopamine, is administered because it can cross the blood-brain barrier, but dopamine cannot.

469. The answer is e. (*Boron, pp 370–372. Guyton, pp 638–640.*) The precentral gyrus is the motor area of the cortex that contains the cell bodies of the neurons that form the corticospinal tract (also referred to as the pyramidal tract). The corticospinal tract contains axons that cross to the contralateral side of the brain within the pyramids and end within the motor areas of the spinal cord. These structures are essential for the generation of fine voluntary movements. Kinesthesia, the sense of movement and position of the limbs, is handled primarily by the Ia and Ib afferents that innervated the muscle spindles and Golgi tendon organs, respectively, and by the parietal lobe.

470. The answer is a. (*Guyton, pp 655–656.*) Ataxia, dysmetria, and an intention tremor all are classic findings in a patient with a lesion involving the cerebellum. Affected persons also exhibit adiadochokinesia, which is a loss of ability to accomplish a swift succession of oscillatory movements, such as moving a finger rapidly up and down. These symptoms all result from destruction of the normal feedback mechanisms that are coordinated in the cerebellum.

471. The answer is b. (*Boron, pp 345–347. Guyton, pp 641–644.*) The otolith organs provide information about the position of the head with respect to gravity. When the head is bent away from its normal upright position, otoliths (small calcium carbonate crystals within the utricle and saccule) are pulled downward by gravity. The crystals bend the stereocilia on the hair cells, causing the hair cells to depolarize. Depolarization of the hair cells stimulates the vestibular nerve fibers. Bending the head in different directions causes different otoliths to move. Therefore, the particular group of vestibular nerve fibers that is stimulated signals the direction in which the head bends.

472. The answer is c. (*Boron, pp 347–340. Guyton, pp 579–581.*) The light-sensitive chemical in the retinal rods is called rhodopsin. It is a combination of 11-cis retinal and opsin. The photoisomerization of 11-cis retinal to all-trans retinal activates rhodopsin. The subsequent separation of opsin and retinal and the reformation of 11-cis rhodopsin are not necessary for the activation of the visual receptors. However, rhodopsin cannot absorb another photon of light until it is enzymatically isomerized back to its 11-cis conformation.

473. The answer is d. (*Boron, pp 402–404. Guyton, pp 711–714.*) The concentrations of protein and glucose within the cerebrospinal fluid (CSF) are much lower than those of plasma. Changes in the CSF concentrations of these substances are helpful in detecting pathologic processes, such as tumor or infection, in which the blood-brain barrier is disrupted. Cerebrospinal fluid, which is in osmotic equilibrium with the extracellular fluid of the brain and spinal cord, is formed primarily in the choroid plexus by an active secretory process. It circulates through the subarachnoid space between the dura mater and pia mater and is absorbed into the circulation by the arachnoid villi. The epidural space, which lies outside the dura mater, may be used clinically for instillation of anesthetics.

474. The answer is b. (*Guyton, pp 674–676.*) When the head rotates in one direction, the hair cells mounted on the cristae rotate along with the head. However, the flow of endolymph is delayed and as a result the cupula is moved in a direction opposite to the movement of the head. When the head moves to the right, the cupula moves toward the left; this bends the stereocilia on the hair cells in the right horizontal canal toward the kinocilium and bends the stereocilia on the hair cells in the left horizontal canal toward the kinocilium. As a result, the hair cells in the right horizontal canal depolarize and those in the left horizontal canal hyperpolarize. The depolarization of the hair cells in the right horizontal canal stimulates the right vestibular nerve, which in turn causes the eyes to deviate toward the left. The movement of the eyes toward the left as the head deviates toward the right keeps the image on the retina in focus.

475. The answer is c. (*Boron, pp 342–343. Guyton, pp 74–78.*) During normal reflex or voluntary movements, small spinal motoneurons are recruited before large motoneurons. Small spinal motoneurons innervate small, weak, slow, fatigue-resistant muscle fibers. Large spinal motoneurons innervate large, fast, strong, easily fatigable muscle fibers. The fatigue-resistant muscle fibers have a dense capillary network for perfusion and use mitochondrial oxidative metabolism to produce ATP.

476. The answer is b. (*Boron, p 733. Guyton, pp 689–691.*) In a normal sleep cycle, a person passes through the four stages of slow-wave sleep before entering REM sleep. In narcolepsy, a person may pass directly from the waking state to REM sleep. REM sleep is characterized by irregular heart beats and respiration and by periods of atonia (loss of muscle tone). Hypoventilation is characteristic of both REM and non-REM sleep because sleep depresses the central chemoreceptors. Brain activity during REM sleep is higher than during wakefulness so there is an increase in brain metabolism. It is also the state of sleep in which dreaming occurs.

477. The answer is d. (*Boron, p 334. Guyton, p 570.*) The increase in lens power that normally occurs when objects are placed close to the eye (the accommodation reflex) does not take place in presbyopia. The failure of the accommodation reflex occurs because the lens and lens capsule stiffen with age. There are some reports of ciliary muscle weakness accompanying presbyopia but there are none indicating the presbyopia is caused by ciliary muscle paralysis.

478. The answer is a. (*Boron, pp 347–340. Guyton, pp 581–582.*) Transducin is the G protein activated by rhodopsin when light strikes the eye. Transducin activates a phosphodiesterase that hydrolyzes cGMP. When cGMP concentrations within the rods or cones decrease, sodium channels close, sodium conductance decreases, and the cell membrane potential increases (hyperpolarizes). Hyperpolarization of the cell causes a decrease in the release of neurotransmitter. Eventually the all-trans retinal dissociates from opsin and reduces the concentration of rhodopsin in the cell.

479. The answer is d. (*Guyton, pp 639–641.*) Spasticity results from overactivity of the alpha motoneurons innervating the skeletal musculature. Under normal circumstances, these alpha motoneurons are tonically stimulated by reticulospinal and vestibulospinal fibers originating in the brainstem. These brainstem fibers are normally inhibited by fibers originating in the cortex. Cutting the cortical fibers releases the brainstem fibers from inhibition and results in spasticity. Cutting the fibers from the reticular formation, vestibular nuclei, or the Ia afferents will reduce the spasticity.

480. The answer is a. (*Boron, pp 347–340. Guyton, pp 581–582.*) Transducin is the G protein that mediates the response to light by rods and cones in the eye. When transducin is activated, it activates an enzyme that hydrolyzes cyclic GMP (cGMP). In the dark, cGMP binds to Na^+ channels, keeping them open. The flow of Na^+ through these channels keeps the rods and cones depolarized. The activation of transducin by light and the subsequent hydrolysis of cGMP cause the Na^+ channels to close and the membrane to hyperpolarize. Hyperpolarization of the membrane prevents the release of an inhibitory transmitter by the rods and cones, which ultimately results in stimulation of optic nerve fibers and the awareness of a visual image.

481. The answer is b. *(Guyton, p 655.)* The flocculonodular lobe is known as the archeocerebellum because it is, phylogenetically, the oldest portion of the cerebellum. It is connected to the vestibular nuclei and participates in the control of eye movements. Lesions to the flocculonodular lobe will cause nystagmus. Lesions to the other regions of the cortex, the deep nuclei of the spinocerebellar tracts, cause a variety of abnormalities in motor coordination referred to as ataxia.

482. The answer is b. *(Guyton, pp 691–692.)* In a totally relaxed adult with eyes closed, the major component of the electroencephalogram (EEG) will be a regular pattern of 8 to 12 waves per second, called the alpha rhythm. The alpha rhythm disappears when the eyes are opened. It is most prominent in the parieto-occipital region. In deep sleep, the alpha rhythm is replaced by larger, slower waves called delta waves. In REM sleep, the EEG will show fast, irregular activity.

483–484. The answers are 483-a, 484-e. *(Boron, pp 70–73, 332–334. Guyton, pp 570–575.)* The focal length of an ideal refractive surface is equal to the distance between the refractive surface and the image formed by a distant object. In a normal eye, the image of a distant object is formed on the retina. Therefore, the focal length is 14 mm. If the image is formed in front of the retina, the eye would be myopic (near-sighted); if the image formed behind the retina, the eye would be hyperopic (far-sighted). When an image is placed close to the eye (in ophthalmology, close means less than 20 ft or 6 m), the eye must accommodate (increase its refractive power) for near vision. The refractive power of a lens system in diopters is equal to the reciprocal of the focal length $(1/f)$ in meters. The relationship between the refractive power P, or focal distance, the image distance, and the object distance is given by the lens formula

$$P = 1/f = 1/o + 1/i$$

where each of the distances is given in meters. If the object distance is 0.25 m and the image distance, the distance from the cornea to the retina, is 0.014 m, the refractive power of the eye is 75 diopters. The initial refractive power was 71 diopters (1/0.014). Therefore, to form a clear image of the object on the retina, the accommodation reflex for near vision increased the refractive power of the eye by 4 diopters.

485. The answer is a. *(Boron, pp 362–363. Guyton, pp 625–626, 628.)* The Ib afferents innervating the quadriceps muscles are activated when the quadriceps contracted in response to tapping the patella tendon. Stretching the patella tendon stretches the intrafusal muscle fibers within the quadriceps muscle and causes an increase in Ia afferent activity. The increase in Ia afferent activity causes an increase in alpha motoneuron activity, which results in contraction of the quadriceps muscle. When the muscle contracts, the intrafusal muscle fibers are unloaded and the Ia afferent activity is reduced.

486. The answer is d. *(Guyton, p 660.)* Huntington's chorea is an inherited genetic defect leading to the degeneration of neurons with the striatum (the caudate nucleus and putamen). It is progressive disease characterized by uncontrolled movements, irritability, depression, and ultimately dementia and death. Lesions of the subthalamic nucleus produce wild flinging movements called ballism; those within the anterior cerebellum produce ataxia; those within the substantia nigra produce Parkinson's disease; and those within the limbic system yield emotional disorders

487. The answer is d. *(Boron, pp 382, 385–387. Guyton, pp 701–703.)* The catecholamines norepinephrine and epinephrine will activate both α- and β-adrenergic receptors. When the α_1-adrenergic receptors are stimulated, they activate a G protein, which in turn activates phospholipase C, which hydrolyzes PIP_2 and produces IP_3 and DAG. The IP_3 causes the release of Ca^{2+} from the sarcoplasmic reticulum, which in turn increases muscle contraction. α_1-adrenergic receptors predominate on arteriolar smooth muscle, so these muscles contract when stimulated with norepinephrine. The bronchiolar, pupillary, and ciliary smooth muscles all contain beta receptors, which cause smooth muscle relaxation. The intestinal smooth muscle relaxation is initiated by an α_2-adrenergic receptor.

488. The answer is e. *(Guyton, pp 607–608.)* A decibel is a measure of the ratio between two sound stimuli. The decibel level of a sound stimulus is referenced to the lowest sound that a normal human can hear and is calculated using the formula: Intensity (in decibels) = 20 × log (sound/threshold). Therefore, the intensity of a sound that is 1000 times threshold is 60 decibels. If the threshold for hearing increases by 1000 times, that is, if the sound intensity must be increased 1000 times for the person with the hearing loss to detect its presence, then the hearing loss is 60 decibels.

489. The answer is a. (*Boron, pp 348–352. Guyton, pp 604–607.*) The portion of the basilar membrane vibrated by a sound depends on the frequency of the sound. High-frequency sounds produce a vibration of the basilar membrane at the base of the cochlea (near the oval and round windows); low-frequency sounds produce a vibration of the basilar membrane at the apex of the cochlea (near the helicotrema). The modiolus is the bony center of the cochlea from which the basilar membrane emerges, the spiral ganglion contains the cell bodies of the auditory nerve fibers, and the stria vascularis is the vascular bed located on the outer wall of the scala media of the cochlea responsible for endolymph secretion.

490. The answer is e. (*Boron, pp 273–275. Guyton, pp 636–639.*) The Babinski reflex causes the toes to dorsiflex in response to stroking the plantar or lateral portion of the foot. It is an abnormal reflex caused by damage to the corticospinal (pyramidal) tract that travels from the cortical motor cortex through the pyramids to the spinal cord. Other signs of pyramidal tract lesions include loss of the hopping and placing reaction, the cremasteric reflex, and the abdominal scratch reflex. Damage confined to the pyramidal tract results in distal muscular weakness and loss of fine motor control. Damage to other areas of the cortical motor control system is referred to as upper motor neuron disease and produces spasticity. Damage to the basal ganglia produces a variety of signs including dystonia (striatum), ballism (subthalamic nucleus), and tremor (substantia nigra). Damaging the cerebellum causes uncoordinated movements (dysmetria).

491. The answer is e. (*Boron, p 1067. Guyton, pp 879–880.*) A variety of physiological functions, such as alertness (the sleep-wake cycle), body temperature, and secretion of hormones, exhibits cyclic activity that varies over a 24-h period of time. These variations in activity are called circadian rhythms and are controlled by the suprachiasmatic nucleus of the hypothalamus. The paraventricular nucleus secretes oxytocin and vasopressin, the ventromedial and lateral nuclei control food intake, and the arcuate nucleus secretes gonadotropin-releasing hormone.

492. The answer is a. (*Guyton, pp 516–517, 523.*) Presynaptic inhibition is caused by interneurons that secrete a transmitter that increases the Cl^- conductance of the presynaptic nerve ending. The increase in Cl^- conductance causes a partial depolarization of the presynaptic nerve ending and a decrease in the magnitude of the action potential in the presynaptic nerve ending. Because the number of synaptic vesicles released from the presynaptic neuron is proportional to the magnitude of the action potential, fewer vesicles are released and magnitude of the postsynaptic potential is reduced. Reducing the magnitude of the postsynaptic potential decreases the probability that an action potential will be generated by the postsynaptic cell. Presynaptic inhibition does not change the membrane potential of the alpha motoneuron.

493. The answer is c. (*Guyton, pp 624–628.*) The firing of the alpha motoneurons to the biceps muscle produces rapid flexion of the arm. Because the arm is rapidly flexed, the Ia afferent neurons innervating the muscle spindles in the biceps, which detect muscle length, will reduce their firing rate. The Ib afferents, innervating the Golgi tendon organs (GTO) from the biceps, will detect the contractile activity of the biceps and increase their firing rate. The triceps are stretched during the arm flexion and so their Ia afferents will increase their firing rate. Ib afferents do not respond when muscles are passively stretched, so their firing rate will not change.

494. The answer is c. (*Boron, pp 392–393, 579–581. Guyton, pp 705–707.*) The entire sympathetic nervous system is activated when a person is frightened, preparing the individual for flight or to fight. As part of this preparation, the smooth muscle of the airways is relaxed, increasing the airway diameter, making it easier for the person to breathe. At the same time, heart rate and cardiac output are increased, causing a rise in blood pressure, and blood glucose concentrations are increased, making fuel available for whatever choice is made.

495. The answer is d. (*Guyton, pp 592, 595–596.*) The optical field defect is produced by an enlarged pituitary gland, which impinges on the optic chiasm. Compression of the optic chiasm by the pituitary gland damages the nasal portion of each optic nerve, which produces a loss of vision in the temporal visual field of both eyes. This defect is referred to as a bitemporal hemianopsia. The pituitary gland hypertrophy is caused by an increased synthesis of thyroid-stimulating hormone (TSH) in response to the decreased circulating thyroxine.

496. The answer is e. (*Guyton, pp 592, 595–596.*) A loss of vision on one side of the visual field is called an hemianopsia. If it affects the same half of the visual field on both eyes, it is called a homonomous hemianopsia. A right-sided homonomous hemianopsia is caused by a lesion affecting the left visual pathway distal to the optic chiasm, where the visual information from the nasal portion of the left retina (the right hemifield of the left eye's visual field) and the temporal portion of the right retina (the right hemifield of the right eye's visual field) are carried within the same nerve tract.

497. The answer is e. (*Boron, pp 356–357. Guyton, pp 552–555.*) Activating nociceptors on the free nerve endings of C fibers produces ischemic pain. The C fibers synapse on interneurons located within the substantia gelatinosa (laminas II and III) of the dorsal horn of the spinal cord. The pathway conveying ischemic pain to the brain is called the paleospinothalamic system. In contrast, well-localized pain sensations are carried within the neospinothalamic tract. Ischemic pain does not adapt to prolonged stimulation. Pain is produced by specific nociceptors and not by intense stimulation of other mechanical, thermal, or chemical receptors.

498. The answer is e. (*Boron, pp 1236–1240. Guyton, pp 826–830.*) The hypothalamus regulates body temperature. Core body temperature, the temperature of the deep tissues of the body, is detected by thermoreceptors located within the anterior hypothalamus. The anterior hypothalamus also contains neurons responsible for initiating reflexes, such as vasodilation and sweating, which are designed to reduce body temperature. Heat-producing reflexes, such as shivering, and head maintenance reflexes, such as vasoconstriction, are initiated by neurons located within the posterior hypothalamus.

499. The answer is a. (*Boron, p 337. Guyton, pp 581–582.*) The visual receptor cells, the rods and cones, are depolarized when the eyes are in the dark. When exposed to light, they hyperpolarize. Light causes the rods and cones to hyperpolarize by activating a G protein called transducin, which leads to the closing of Na^+ channels. Auditory receptors are depolarized by the flow of K^+ into the hair cells. Touch receptors are activated by opening channels through which both Na^+ and K^+ can flow. Depolarization is caused by the inward flow of Na^+. Smell and taste receptors are activated by

G protein–mediated mechanisms, some of which cause the receptor cell to depolarize; other G proteins cause the release of synaptic transmitter without any change in membrane potential.

500. The answer is a. *(Guyton, pp 686–687.)* The Klüver-Bucy syndrome is produced in animals by removal of the amygdala from both temporal lobes. The syndrome is characterized by a tendency to examine objects orally and excessive sexual behavior. The full syndrome is rarely encountered in humans but many of its characteristics are observed in patients with bilateral temporal lobe lesions produced by encephalitis or traumatic injury.

Bibliography

Boron WF, Boulpaep EL: *Medical Physiology*. Philadelphia, WB Saunders, 2003.

Guyton AC, Hall MN: *Textbook of Medical Physiology*, 10/e. Philadelphia, WB Saunders, 2000.

Index